Curbside
Consultation
in Neuro-Ophthalmology

49 Clinical Questions

CURBSIDE CONSULTATION IN OPHTHALMOLOGY

SERIES

SERIES EDITOR, DAVID F. CHANG, MD

Curbside Consultation
in Neuro-Ophthalmology

49 Clinical Questions

Editor

Andrew G. Lee, MD
Professor of Ophthalmology, Neurology, and Neurosurgery
H. Stanley Thompson Neuro-ophthalmology Clinic
University of Iowa Hospitals and Clinics
Iowa City, Iowa

Associate Editors

Paul W. Brazis, MD
Consultant in Neurology and Neuro-Ophthalmology
Professor of Neurology
Mayo Clinic—Jacksonville
Jacksonville, Florida

Lanning B. Kline, MD
Professor and Chair
Department of Ophthalmology
University of Alabama School of Medicine
Birmingham, Alabama

SLACK
INCORPORATED
Delivering the best in health care information and education worldwide

ISBN: 978-1-55642-840-1

Published by: SLACK Incorporated
                 6900 Grove Road
                 Thorofare, NJ 08086 USA
                 Telephone: 856-848-1000
                 Fax: 856-848-6091
                 www.slackbooks.com

Contact SLACK Incorporated for more information about other books in this field or about the availability of our books from distributors outside the United States.

Library of Congress Cataloging-in-Publication Data

Curbside consultation in neuro-ophthalmology : 49 clinical questions / edited by Andrew G. Lee, Paul W. Brazis, Lanning B. Kline.
    p. ; cm. -- (Curbside consultation in ophthalmology)
  Includes bibliographical references and index.
  ISBN 978-1-55642-840-1 (alk. paper)
  1. Neuroophthalmology--Miscellanea. I. Lee, Andrew G. II. Brazis, Paul W. III. Kline, Lanning B. IV. Series: Curbside consultation in ophthalmology series.
  [DNLM: 1. Optic Nerve Diseases--diagnosis. 2. Optic Nerve Diseases--therapy. WW 280 C975 2008]
  RE725.C868 2008
  617.7'32--dc22
                              2008025266

Printed in the United States of America.

Last digit is print number: 10   9   8   7   6   5   4   3   2   1

Dedication

I would like to dedicate this book to my brother, Richard Lee, and to my sister, Amy Wirts, MD, who taught me the value of a quick curbside opinion not just in medicine but for life's questions in general. I also thank my wonderful parents, Rosalind Lee, MD and Alberto Lee, MD, for teaching me the importance of asking for help and giving help when needed. I also recognize the invaluable and unwavering support of my wife, Hilary Beaver, MD, and hope that my 2 children, Rachael Lee and Virginia Lee, will one day follow the long line of white coats into the profession of medicine.

Andrew G. Lee, MD

I would like to thank my parents, Dr. and Mrs. Peter T. Brazis, who have helped me throughout my life and medical career. I would especially like to acknowledge and express his appreciation to my family, including Elizabeth, Erica, Paul, and Kelly Brazis, and now also the newest member of the Brazis family, Hannah. I would also like to express special thanks to the late Dr. Frank Rubino, whose teaching abilities, compassion, and concern for patients will be truly missed by future students, residents, and clinicians.

Paul W. Brazis, MD

I dedicate this book to my colleagues, both established practitioners and residents-in-training. They continue to "keep me on my toes" by challenging me with questions regarding diagnosis and therapy. Each patient with a neuro-ophthalmic disorder is unique and must be approached carefully and thoughtfully. I hope the reader will find this text valuable; it emphasizes the art as well as the science of neuro-ophthalmology.

Lanning B. Kline, MD

Contents

About the Editor

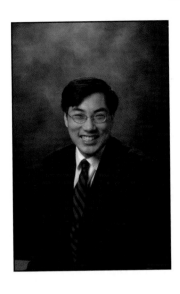

Andrew G. Lee, MD is a graduate of the University of Virginia undergraduate school and the School of Medicine. He completed his ophthalmology residency and was the chief resident at Baylor College of Medicine in Houston, TX in 1993. Following his residency, Dr. Lee completed a fellowship in neuro-ophthalmology with Neil R. Miller, MD at the Wilmer Ophthalmological Institute and was a postdoctoral Fight for Sight fellow at the Johns Hopkins Hospital in Baltimore, MD from 1993 to 1994. He was formerly an Associate Professor at Baylor College of Medicine and Adjunct Associate Professor at the MD Anderson Cancer Center in Houston from 1994 to 2000. He has published over 260 peer-reviewed articles, 40 book chapters, and 2 full textbooks in ophthalmology. Dr. Lee serves on the editorial board of 12 journals, including the *American Journal of Ophthalmology*, the *Canadian Journal of Ophthalmology*, and *Eye*. He has received the American Academy of Ophthalmology (AAO) Honor Award, the AAO Secretariat Award, and the AAO Senior Achievement Award. He has been the invited guest or visiting professor at over 150 medical meetings. Dr. Lee is currently Professor of Ophthalmology, Neurology, and Neurosurgery in the H. Stanley Thompson Neuro-Ophthalmology Clinic at the University of Iowa Hospitals and Clinics.

About the Associate Editors

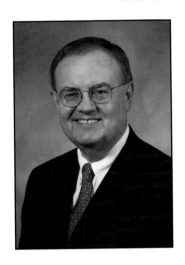

Paul W. Brazis, MD received his undergraduate degree from the University of Notre Dame and his medical degree from Loyola University–Stritch School of Medicine. After his medical internship at Presbyterian-St. Lukes Hospital in Chicago, he returned to Loyola University-Stritch School of Medicine for a neurology residency. His fellowship in Neuro-Ophthalmology was at Johns Hopkins Medical Center-Wilmer Ophthalmological Institute in Baltimore.

Dr. Brazis is presently a Professor of Neurology in the Mayo Clinic School of Medicine and a consultant in neurology and neuro-ophthalmology for the Mayo Clinic at Jacksonville. He was voted the Outstanding Faculty Member in 1999, 2001, and 2002 for his lectures with the Mayo Clinic School of Continuing Medical Education and received the Distinguished Mayo Clinician Award for the Jacksonville Mayo Clinic in 2001. He has co-authored several texts in neurology and neuro-ophthalmology. One of his textbooks, *Localization in Clinical Neurology*, is now in its fifth edition.

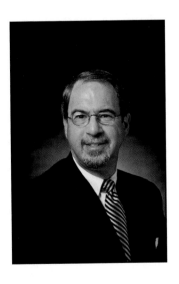

Lanning B. Kline, MD is a native of Edmonton, Alberta, Canada. He received his bachelor of arts degree from the University of Alberta and graduated from Duke University School of Medicine. He served an internship at Duke University Department of Ophthalmology and a residency in the Department of Ophthalmology, McGill University, Montreal, Quebec, Canada. Dr. Kline completed fellowships in neuro-ophthalmology at the Montreal Neurological Institute and at the Bascom Palmer Eye Institute, Miami, FL.

Dr. Kline has been a faculty member in the UAB Department of Ophthalmology since 1979. In 1998, he became Professor and Chairman of the department, and in 2000 was appointed to the EyeSight Foundation of Alabama Endowed Chair in Ophthalmology.

Dr. Kline is certified by the American Board of Ophthalmology, is a member of the North American Neuro-Ophthalmology Society, and is a Fellow of the American College of Surgeons.

Contributing Authors

Laura J. Balcer, MD, MSCE (Question 15)
University of Pennsylvania
Philadelphia, PA

M. Tariq Bhatti, MD (Question 7)
Duke University Eye Center
Durham, NC

Valérie Biousse, MD (Question 23)
Emory University School of Medicine
Emory Eye Center
Atlanta, GA

Mark Borchert, MD (Question 1)
Vision Center at Childrens Hospital Los
Angeles
USC/Keck School of Medicine
Los Angeles, CA

Swaraj Bose, MD (Question 27)
University of California
Irvine, CA
Cedars-Sinai Medical Center
Los Angeles, CA

Thomas J. Carlow, MD (Question 39)
University of New Mexico, School of
Medicine
Eye Associates of New Mexico
Albuquerque, NM

Pamela S. Chavis, MD (Question 16)
Medical University South Carolina
Storm Eye Institute
Charleston, SC

Sophia M. Chung, MD (Question 21)
Saint Louis University School of Medicine
St. Louis, MO

Kimberly Cockerham, MD (Question 19)
Stanford University
Los Altos, CA

James J. Corbett, MD (Question 32)
University of Mississippi Medical Center
Jackson, MS

Wayne T. Cornblath, MD (Question 33)
University of Michigan
Ann Arbor, MI

Fiona Costello, MD, FRCP (Question 3)
University of Calgary
Calgary, Alberta, Canada

Kathleen B. Digre, MD (Question 28)
Moran Eye Center
University of Utah
Salt Lake City, UT

Drew Dixon, MD (Question 13)
University of Colorado Denver School of
Medicine
Denver, CO

Eric Eggenberger, DO, MSEpi (Question 4)
Michigan State University
East Lansing, MI

Julie Falardeau, MD, FRCSC (Question 26)
Casey Eye Institute—Oregon Health and
Science University and Devers Eye Institute
Portland, OR

Steven E. Feldon, MD, MBA (Question 18)
University of Rochester School of Medicine
& Dentristry
University of Rochester Eye Institute
Rochester, NY

Rod Foroozan, MD (Question 6)
Baylor College of Medicine
Houston, Texas

Deborah I. Friedman, MD, FAAN (Question 12)
University of Rochester School of Medicine and Dentistry
Rochester, NY

Steven L. Galetta, MD (Question 5)
Hospital of the University of Pennsylvania
Philadelphia, PA

James A. Garrity, MD (Question 17)
Mayo Clinic
College of Medicine
Rochester, MN

Christopher C. Glisson, DO (Question 14)
Michigan State University
East Lansing, MI
Saint Mary's Health Care
Grand Rapids, MI

Karl C. Golnik, MD, MEd (Question 29)
University of Cincinnati and the Cincinnati Eye Institute
Cincinnati, OH

Jennifer K. Hall, MD (Question 10)
University of Pennsylvania
Philadelphia, PA

Steven R. Hamilton, MD (Question 41)
University of Washington
Neuro-ophthalmic Consultants Northwest
Seattle, WA

Andrew R. Harrison, MD (Question 44)
University of Minnesota
Minneapolis, MN

Jonathan C. Horton, MD, PhD (Question 36)
Beckman Vision Center
University of California, San Francisco
San Francisco, CA

Thomas N. Hwang, MD, PhD (Question 43)
University of California, San Francisco
San Francisco, CA

Randy Kardon, MD, PhD (Question 24)
University of Iowa Hospital and Clinics & Veterans Administration
Iowa City, IA

David I. Kaufman, DO (Question 14)
Michigan State University
East Lansing, MI

Aki Kawasaki, MD (Question 25)
Médécin-Associée
Hôpital Ophtalmique Jules Gonin
University of Lausanne
Lausanne, Switzerland

Melissa W. Ko, MD (Question 5)
State University of New York at Upstate Medical University
Syracuse, NY

Greg Kosmorsky, DO (Question 42)
Cleveland Clinic
Cleveland, OH

Byron L. Lam, MD (Question 35)
Bascom Palmer Eye Institute
University of Miami
Miami, FL

Jacqueline A. Leavitt, MD (Question 9)
Mayo Clinic
Rochester, MN

Michael S. Lee, MD (Question 44)
University of Minnesota
Minneapolis, MN

Robert L. Lesser, MD *(Question 45)*
Yale University School of Medicine
New Haven, CT
University of Connecticut School of Medicine
Farmington, CT

Leah Levi, MBBS *(Question 47)*
Shiley Eye Center
University of California, San Diego
San Diego, CA

Grant T. Liu, MD *(Question 30)*
University of Pennsylvania School of Medicine
Hospital of the University of Pennsylvania
Children's Hospital of Philadelphia
Philadelphia, PA

Timothy J. McCulley, MD *(Question 43)*
University of California, San Francisco
San Francisco, CA

Neil R. Miller, MD *(Question 2)*
Johns Hopkins Medical Institutions
Baltimore, MD

Gautam R. Mirchandani, MD *(Question 37)*
Columbia University College of Physicians and Surgeons
New York, NY

Nancy J. Newman, MD *(Question 48)*
Emory University School of Medicine
Atlanta, GA
Harvard Medical School
Cambridge, MA

Steve Newman, MD *(Question 31)*
University of Virginia Health Science Center
Charlottesville, VA

Jeffrey Odel, MD *(Question 37)*
Edward S. Harkness Eye Institute
Columbia University College of Physicians and Surgeons
New York, NY

Sang-Rog Oh, MD *(Question 37)*
Edward S. Harkness Eye Institute
Columbia University College of Physicians and Surgeons
New York, NY

Victoria S. Pelak, MD *(Question 13)*
University of Colorado Denver School of Medicine and The Denver Veterans Affairs Medical Center
Denver, CO

Raymond Price, MD *(Question 15)*
University of Pennsylvania
Philadelphia, PA

Janet C. Rucker, MD *(Question 20)*
Rush University
Chicago, IL

Alfredo A. Sadun, MD, PhD *(Question 8)*
Doheny Eye Institute
University of Southern California—Keck School of Medicine
Los Angeles, CA

Peter Savino, MD *(Question 16)*
Wills Eye Institute
Philadelphia, PA

Robert H. Spector, MD *(Question 46)*
Neuro-ophthalmology
Atlanta, GA

Madhura A. Tamhankar, MD *(Question 30)*
Scheie Eye Institute
University of Pennsylvania School of Medicine
Philadelphia, PA

Rosa Ana Tang, MD, MPH (Question 34)
University of Texas Health Science Center
Houston, TX
MS Eye CARE—University Eye Institute
Houston, TX

Matthew J. Thurtell, MBBS, FRACP (Question 40)
University Hospitals Case Medical Center
Cleveland, OH

Robert L. Tomsak, MD, PhD (Question 40)
University Hospitals Case Medical Center
Cleveland, OH

Roger Turbin, MD (Question 49)
University of Medicine and Dentistry, New
Jersey Medical School
Newark, NJ

Michael S. Vaphiades, DO (Question 38)
University of Alabama at Birmingham
Birmingham, AL

Nicholas J. Volpe, MD (Question 10)
Scheie Eye Institute University of Penn-
sylvania
Philadelphia, PA

Michael Wall, MD (Question 11)
University of Iowa College of Medicine
Veterans Administration Hospital
Iowa City, IA

Brian R. Younge, MD (Question 22)
Mayo Clinic
Rochester, MN

Preface

The informal consult (ie, the "curbside consult") is a common and indispensable part of the practice of medicine. The busy clinician faced with a diagnostic or treatment dilemma can solicit practical advice from a knowledgeable expert in a short period of time. Every day across the United States and the world, these brief curbside consultations are taking place in clinic hallways, over the telephone, at lunch, or nowadays by email. The question is typically brief and concise. The advice is practical, to the point, and based upon that expert's knowledge, judgment, and experience. It is the essence of the "curbside consult" that this book wishes to capture.

Curbside Consultation in Neuro-Ophthalmology is part of a larger series of textbooks being developed for ophthalmologists by SLACK Incorporated. The series' goal is to provide a compendium of this type of clinical information—answers to the thorny questions most commonly posed to specialists by residents and practicing colleagues. We hope that this educational question-and-answer–type format will be unique among the available publications in ophthalmology.

We have compiled 49 questions and posed them to a master clinician in the field. The clinical advice is based upon personal experience but supported by the evidence-based literature. The answers to the curbside questions are designed to meet 4 criteria of content—the 4 "C's"—current (timely), concise (summarizing), credible (evidence based), and clinically relevant (practical).

The primary target audience for this book is the practicing ophthalmologist. Although we hope the information will be simple enough to help residents and fellows in training, the goal is to provide current and concise advice for a clinician who already has some knowledge of the field.

Where possible, we try to use the first person—"You first need to stop and do this" and "I prefer doing using this"—and we are intentionally avoiding a lengthy or formal review of the literature.

We recognize that the management of many of these clinical problems will be controversial, and we emphasize to the reader that the curbside opinions and preferences of the authors represent the individual author's viewpoint based upon his or her clinical experience and should not be misinterpreted as a standard of care or a hard and fast rule for every situation.

We hope that you will enjoy reading this book as much as we enjoyed putting it together.

Andrew G. Lee, MD
Paul W. Brazis, MD
Lanning B. Kline, MD

How Should a Childhood Optic Nerve Glioma Be Worked Up?

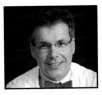

Mark Borchert, MD

An 8-year-old boy presents with vision of 20/40 right eye (OD) and 20/20 left eye (OS). He has a right relative afferent pupillary defect (RAPD) and a pale optic nerve OD. The left fundus is normal. Magnetic resonance imaging (MRI) findings are consistent with a right optic nerve glioma. How should this patient be evaluated?

Let us be frank. There are no treatments with demonstrated effectiveness in curing optic gliomas or preventing the vision loss that may be associated with them. Thus, the main management decision is determining if and when the various unproven and in some cases even somewhat "experimental" therapy should be started. This decision depends on understanding the prognosis for untreated optic nerve gliomas, which in turn, depends on the age of the patient and whether or not he or she is afflicted with neurofibromatosis type 1 (NF-1).

In general, patients with NF-1 have a better visual prognosis and their optic nerve gliomas rarely cause progressive vision loss beyond the age of 12. An assessment of afflicted children for café-au-lait spots, Lisch nodules, and family history of possible NF-1 is essential. Genotyping is rarely necessary but is available and should be discussed with a geneticist. You should be more reluctant to pull the treatment trigger on a patient with NF-1, since the untreated prognosis is relatively good, and since there is a theoretical risk of inducing tumors elsewhere in patients with a mutation of a growth control gene. This is of particular concern if your oncologist is considering radiation therapy.

Regardless of whether or not the afflicted patient has NF-1, I believe that no treatment should be started without documented progression of vision loss or hypothalamic dysfunction. The fact that the patient presents with diminished vision is not sufficient. The diminished vision may have been stable for years, even for life. It is also not sufficient for a single decrement in visual acuity from one exam to the next to be considered progressive vision loss. Many patients have fluctuating vision or full recovery of vision regardless of whether or not the tumor is changing in size on the MRI scan. Consequently, there should be some documentation of progressive vision loss over at least 2 to 3 examinations and the vision loss should be approaching the threshold for a change in functional significance (eg, losing reading ability or independent mobility).

Since your particular patient is 8 years old and literate age, you have many monitoring tools at your disposal to help in your decision as to when to refer for chemotherapy. Besides measuring best-corrected visual acuity, you can monitor visual fields. This is best done with Goldmann perimetry, since it is more reliable than automated perimetry at this age and since the examiner can focus on those areas of known field loss before the patient's attention is lost. You should also consider monitoring color vision. I would not base treatment decisions on color vision, but an isolated drop in color vision would cause me to increase the examination frequency. Finally, baseline optic disc photos and/or optical coherence tomography should be obtained and repeated for confirmation if there is suspicion of worsening optic atrophy.

How often should you follow this patient? In general, the frequency of visits depends on the stability of the examination and the age of the patient. The longer you follow a patient with a stable ophthalmic examination, the less frequent need be the visits. I will usually see an 8-year-old patient 2 to 3 months following the first examination, then semi-annually for 2 to 3 years, then annually. I will follow children who present at less than 3 years of age more frequently.

The role of repeat neuroimaging is controversial. I generally do not find it useful in making treatment decisions unless I suspect nonophthalmic consequences of tumor enlargement, such as hypopituitarism or impending hydrocephalus. Nonetheless, parents seem to find comfort in documenting neuroradiographic stability or even shrinkage. Spontaneous regression of optic gliomas with or without improvement in vision has also been documented on serial MRI scans.

As I previously mentioned, the treatment options are limited. Most neuro-oncologists will treat with some combination of chemotherapy that includes vincristine, carboplatin, and/or temozolomide. The side effects of these medications are similar to, but generally less severe than, those used to treat most childhood malignancies. These agents are believed to arrest progression and, in some cases, cause tumor regression based on MRI. No controlled studies and no studies using vision outcomes have been done.

Surgical excision of unilateral optic gliomas has been advocated in some cases to prevent progression to chiasm involvement or to relieve unsightly exophthalmos. Obviously, this treatment causes blindness, so it should probably be reserved for patients with severely impaired vision. The effectiveness of surgical excision is controversial. There is no evidence that optic gliomas actually spread to uninvolved parts of the visual pathways. There have been numerous documented cases of histological involvement of the chiasm despite the fact that the tumor appeared confined to the orbit on MRI scan.

Radiation therapy results in tumor shrinkage but can also cause worsening vision loss. It should best be avoided if possible in very young children because of the concomitant risk of cognitive impairment and hypothalamic injury.

Fortunately, progressive vision loss and nonophthalmic complications are the exception, rather than the rule, in cases such as these. In my experience, parents are relieved to hear this and can accept expectant observation as a management option over immediate treatment once the facts about optic gliomas and their treatment are calmly explained.

Summary

* Optic nerve glioma is typically a tumor of childhood.
* Some patients have NF-1.
* No treatment has been proven to be effective.
* Observation for clinical or radiographic stability or progression is the first line of management.
* Chemotherapy and radiation therapy have been used in selected patients with progressive disease but is unproven.
* Surgical excision of an optic nerve glioma has a limited role for patients with blind eyes with cosmetically unacceptable proptosis.

Bibliography

Hwang JM, Cheon JE, Wang KC. Visual prognosis of optic glioma. *Childs Nerv Syst.* 2008; PMID 18175125.
Parsa CF, Hoyt CS, Lesser RL, et al. Spontaneous regression of optic gliomas: thirteen cases documented by serial neuroimaging. *Arch Ophthalmol.* 2001;119:516-529.

2

HOW SHOULD AN OPTIC NERVE SHEATH MENINGIOMA BE MANAGED?

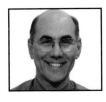

Neil R. Miller, MD

A 50-year-old otherwise healthy woman has had progressive visual loss for 2 years in her right eye. She was scanned and a right optic nerve sheath meningioma on her magnetic resonance imaging (MRI) was found. Her vision is 20/40 OD, and she has a relative afferent pupillary defect (RAPD) and an inferior visual field defect OD. The left eye was normal. The right optic nerve is pale and a retinochoroidal venous collateral on the optic nerve head is seen. What should be done now?

Based on her history, clinical findings, and neuroimaging, your patient has a presumed optic nerve sheath meningioma (ONSM). ONSMs have 3 main morphologic patterns on imaging: 1) tubular, 2) fusiform, and 3) globular. Computed tomography (CT) scanning typically shows enlargement of the optic nerve with an increased density peripherally and decreased density centrally (the "tram-track" sign) (Figure 2-1). These changes are particularly well seen after intravenous injection of iodinated contrast material. In addition, in some cases of ONSM, calcifications surrounding the nerve are present on CT scanning, although they may be masked by contrast enhancement and thus are best identified on precontrast soft-tissue and bone-windowed images. MRI provides somewhat better detail of ONSMs than does CT scanning. In particular, the soft-tissue component of the tumor is readily visible, particularly when T1-weighted images are viewed after intravenous injection of a paramagnetic contrast agent and fat saturation techniques are used. The appearance of the optic nerve on coronal MRI after gadolinium is most often that of a hypodense area (the nerve) surrounded by an enhancing thin, fusiform, or globular peripheral ring of tissue (the tumor) (Figure 2-2). In addition, on careful examination, rather than having a perfectly smooth outline, all forms of ONSMs can be seen to have

Figure 2-1. CT scan, axial view, showing appearance of left ONSM. Note thickening of nerve with "tram-track" sign.

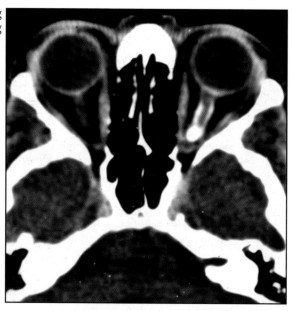

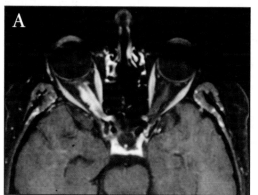
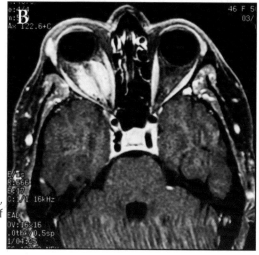

Figure 2-2. MRI, T1-weighted, fat-suppressed, contrast-enhanced axial views in 2 types of ONSM. (A) Diffuse type. (B) Fusiform type.

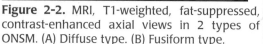

very fine extensions into the orbit (Figure 2-3). MRI also provides sufficient tissue detail that one can use to assess intracranial extension. Ultrasound of the orbit can also be helpful in the diagnosis of an ONSM. Echographic evaluation of an ONSM characteristically shows an enlargement in the diameter of the nerve, with predominantly medium-high reflectivity and an irregular acoustic structure. In addition, you might see shadowing from internal calcification. In many cases, performance of a 30-degree test reveals solid thickening of the nerve, whereas in others, the tumor is located more posteriorly, and the anterior enlargement of the nerve is due to cerebrospinal fluid that is trapped by the tumor. These studies generally obviate the need for tissue biopsy in most cases, making an early diagnosis possible without potentially damaging the optic nerve during surgery. Nevertheless, metastatic infiltration of the optic nerve and optic nerve sheath, as well as lymphoma and inflammatory lesions, such as sarcoid and sclerosing orbital inflamma-

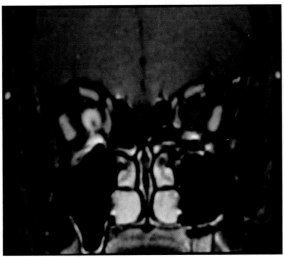

Figure 2-3. MRI, T1-weighted, fat-suppressed, contrast-enhanced coronal view of diffuse type of ONSM. Note enhancing tissue with irregular borders surrounding the right optic nerve, which is the tumor. The nerve itself appears as a small, hypodense central area.

tion, may mimic ONSMs, and these should be considered in the differential diagnosis of a patient with a presumed ONSM. In most cases, the history and clinical setting will suffice to eliminate these other processes.

The first thing for you to remember in managing a patient with a presumed ONSM is that the tumor is not lethal, will not cause a catastrophic neurologic deficit, and is highly unlikely to spread across the planum sphenoidale and cause loss of vision in the opposite eye. Thus, management of a patient with a presumed ONSM should be aimed at restoring or at least preserving visual function in the affected eye. To date, trials of medical therapy for ONSM, such as those using estrogen or progesterone antagonists, have not been successful, and attempts to excise these tumors while keeping the optic nerve itself intact are usually unsuccessful, with most patients becoming blind in the eye following surgery. Indeed, it has been shown that radiation therapy is the only treatment capable of preserving and occasionally improving vision in patients with ONSMs. Several types of radiation therapy have been utilized, including conventional fractionated radiation therapy, stereotactic radiosurgery, and stereotactic fractionated radiation therapy (SFR). Unfortunately, radiation therapy has significant risks. The major concern with radiotherapy for ONSMs is late toxicity. Not only can radiation damage the optic nerve itself, but adjacent tissues can also be damaged, including the retina, pituitary gland, and the white-matter tracts of the brain. Retinal injury may occur, particularly if the tumor extends to the globe and a total dose of more than 50 Gy is used, but coexistence of diabetes mellitus may lower the threshold for retinal or optic nerve damage to 45 Gy. The threshold for radiation damage to the optic nerve has been estimated to be 8 to 10 Gy for a single dose. Because lower doses of radiation are thought to have a more uncertain effect on benign tumors such as ONSMs, and a large, single dose of radiation is associated with a high risk of tissue damage, single-dose stereotactic radiosurgery is not widely used to treat ONSMs. SFR, on the other hand, appears to offer the potential for delivering a sufficient amount of radiation to an ONSM in a manner more focused than that of conventional fractionated radiation therapy, thus minimizing (but not eliminating) the complications from exposure of the surrounding tissue to high doses of radiation.

I would recommend the following. The first step in determining the management of this patient is to determine if your patient feels that her visual loss is sufficient for her to accept the potential risks of radiation that will, in part, be related to the extent of the lesion. If your patient wishes to undergo treatment and accepts its risks, then SFR is the treatment of choice. SFR requires complex planning, which is facilitated by sophisticated software and three-dimensional imaging. The pretreatment imaging (CT and/or MRI) and radiation delivery require the patient to be repeatedly immobilized, although the newest linear accelerator (LINAC) units such as the Cyberknife (Accuray, Sunnyvale, CA) use a tracking system that eliminates the need for rigid immobilization during the treatment phase. Unlike conventional radiation therapy, the LINAC system delivers the radiation in noncoplanar fields that take into account the characteristics of the surrounding tissue. Every beam is size- and shape-adjusted by different devices, micro-leaf collimators being the most advanced way of achieving a high degree of conformality to the tumor, thus minimizing irradiation of the surrounding tissue. Nevertheless, the more extensive the lesion, the more field will have to be covered by the radiation, and the greater the risk of damage to the globe.

I think that your patient may be a candidate for radiation therapy. Let me know how she does.

Summary

* ONSM usually can be diagnosed by clinical and neuroimaging findings.

* SFR is the recommended treatment for patients with ONSM if the goal is stabilization or preservation of vision.

* Surgical excision of ONSM is not generally recommended, and the risk of a primary ONSM spreading to the fellow eye is low.

Bibliography

Andrews DW, Foroozan R, Yang BP, et al. Fractionated stereotactic radiotherapy for the treatment of optic nerve sheath meningiomas: preliminary observations of 33 optic nerves in 30 patients with historical comparison to observation with or without prior surgery. *Neurosurgery.* 2002;51:890-902.

Miller NR. The evolving management of optic nerve sheath meningiomas. *Br J Ophthalmol.* 2002;86:1198.

Miller NR. New concepts in the diagnosis and management of optic nerve sheath meningioma. *J Neuroophthalmol.* 2006;26:200-208.

Subramanian PS, Bressler NM, Miller NR. Radiation retinopathy after fractionated stereotactic radiotherapy for optic nerve sheath meningioma. *Ophthalmology.* 2004;111:565-567.

Turbin RE, Thompson CR, Kennerdell JS, Cockerham KP, Kupersmith MJ. A long-term visual outcome comparison in patients with optic nerve sheath meningioma managed with observation, surgery, radiotherapy, or surgery and radiotherapy. *Ophthalmology.* 2002;109:890-899.

WHAT NEUROIMAGING STUDIES SHOULD I ORDER?

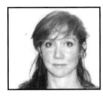

Fiona Costello, MD, FRCP

How do you decide what neuroimaging study to perform for your patients with neuro-oph-thalmic problems? For example, pupil-involved third nerve palsy, unexplained optic atrophy, optic neuritis, nystagmus, orbital or cavernous sinus syndromes, or amaurosis fugax?

That is a great question. Every day I am challenged to answer for my own patients, "What imaging modality is the best one to choose for this patient?" In general, my own answer depends on the following set of questions that I ask myself before I order the study:

* What is the nature of the neuro-ophthalmic problem?
* When do I need this test?
* Who is the patient?
* Where is the lesion likely to be?

What Determines When and When Determines What

The potential urgency of a neuro-ophthalmic problem is paramount to determining your choice of imaging modality because urgent issues require rapid intervention. Therefore, in the case of a potentially vision- or life-threatening prob-

he imaging option that allows you to confirm or refute your clini-
s quickly. In the case of the patient with sudden-onset headache and
an unenhanced computed tomography (CT) scan, with and without
conu.. ovides vital information in a time-efficient manner. Therefore, CT is generally the initial imaging modality of choice in the evaluation of acute infarction,
trauma, or hemorrhage. CT provides rapid information about brain, orbit, and bone and
has the advantages of being readily attainable and cost effective. Associated disadvantag-
es include ionizing radiation, beam-hardening artifacts (from bone and metallic objects),
and iodinated contrast-induced allergic reactions and nephrotoxicity.

Magnetic resonance imaging (MRI) is superior to CT in the evaluation of most neuro-
ophthalmic lesions, except for acute hemorrhage and bony abnormalities. Yet, because
MRI scans can be difficult to obtain after hours, this imaging modality is not ideal for
evaluating urgent neuro-ophthalmic problems. Often, the safest course of action is to
choose a baseline CT scan, and then pursue MRI later, as indicated.

For urgent vascular problems, CT and MR angiography (CTA and MRA) and venography (MRV) techniques offer the advantages of being relatively safe and noninvasive as
compared to the gold standard of digital subtraction angiography (DSA). In the context
of suspected cerebral venous sinus thrombosis (CVST), MRV can provide detailed information about venous integrity, but interpretation requires knowledge of different stages
of thrombus evolution. MRV has the benefit of providing complementary MRI views,
which can detect parenchymal lesions and subtle signs of raised intracranial pressure.
Yet, because computed tomography venography (CTV) can often be obtained faster and
demonstrates fewer equivocal findings than MRV, it is often my first imaging modality
of choice for CVST, particularly in the emergency room setting.

In the case of a pupil-involving third nerve palsy, I would favor a combined cranial
MRI and MRA study in ideal circumstances as the initial study. This combination of
imaging provides detailed views of the vascular anatomy and superior tissue resolution
in the relevant areas of interest, including the cavernous sinus. However, in an emergency
room setting, I would opt instead for a CT and complementary computed tomography
angiography (CTA), both to check for subarachnoid hemorrhage and to detect an intracranial aneurysm. This information can be ascertained very quickly while the patient is
already in the CT scanner. Once the pivotal question about the potentially life-threatening
diagnosis is answered, I can then direct an appropriate clinical management strategy and
make a determination of whether a standard catheter angiogram might still be needed.

Identifying the "Who's Who" of Neuroimaging

Who the patient is plays a major role in your choice of neuroimaging study. CT carries
the risks of ionizing radiation, which makes MRI a more desirable choice for pregnant
patients. Similarly, in patients with significant renal impairment, MRI may be preferable
to CT due to the risk of iodinated contrast-induced nephrotoxicity. Unfortunately, even
with MRI the emergence of a new gadolinium-related condition—nephrogenic systemic
fibrosis—has created new requirements for screening and caution in the use of gadolinium for MRI in patients with renal failure. I would recommend consulting with your
local neuroradiology department for questions of gadolinium use in this setting as the
guidelines are still evolving.

Patient claustrophobia, significant obesity, cardiac pacemakers, and ferromagnetic substances (surgical hardware, dental appliances, and cochlear implants) may contraindicate MRI for some patients. Who the patient is may also prompt me to forgo neuroimaging in certain circumstances. For example, I do not routinely repeat MRI scans for patients with an established diagnosis of multiple sclerosis (MS) who experience relapses because it is costly and clinically unnecessary to do so. I may reimage these patients if I suspect an alternate diagnosis or if my clinical management may change depending on the outcome of the scan. Furthermore, for palliative patients with a poor prognosis for long-term survival, I adhere to the adage "less is more." When the choice of imaging modality is likely to cause the patient discomfort or potential morbidity and provide little benefit to the clinical situation, the best test, in my opinion, is no test at all.

Location, Location, Location...

MRI provides optimal visualization of most neuro-ophthalmic lesions because of its superior tissue resolution in the posterior orbit, chiasm, cavernous sinus, postchiasmal visual pathways, and posterior fossa. As an imaging modality, MRI allows you to obtain multiplanar imaging without patient repositioning. For patients with suspected optic neuritis, baseline MRI features can predict the future risk of MS. In the case of suspected optic neuritis, I like to include views of the orbit, brain, and cervical spine. In this manner I can identify not only the cranial white matter abnormalities predictive of future MS, but also detect the spinal lesions that implicate neuro-myelitis optica as a contending diagnosis. Gadolinium-enhanced MRI provide detailed anatomical information about lesions of the optic nerve (nerve sheath meningiomas, gliomas, sarcoidosis, optic neuritis), orbital apex, and cavernous sinus (meningiomas, pituitary lesions). For imaging of the postchiasmal visual pathways, optimal results can be achieved with axial T1, T2, fluid-attenuated inversion recovery (FLAIR), and diffusion-weighted MR techniques. Gadolinium-enhanced MRI can be used to detect tumors, meningitis, abscess, and demyelination. For patients with oscillopsia or diplopia due to suspected brainstem, cerebellar, and craniocervical junction abnormalities, MRI provides superior views to CT in visualization of the posterior fossa structures. Similarly, for patients with suspected Horner's syndrome, MRI/MRA techniques can allow visualization of lesions involving the sympathetic chain from the hypothalamus to the T1 level of the spinal cord.

MRA (including time of flight and dynamic three-dimensional contrast-enhanced methods) may be performed in concert with conventional MRI to detect diffusion-perfusion mismatch in acute stroke and evolving blood products. MRA is complemented by fat saturation sequences that aid in detection and characterization of dissecting hematomas and pseudoaneurysms in arterial structures. In general, MRA has a sensitivity and specificity similar to CTA for detection of aneurysms that are 5 mm or larger in diameter but may have lower sensitivity for detection of lesions less than 5 mm. The clinical setting in which MRA is superior to CTA is in the assessment of aneurysms previously treated with endovascular coils. Both MRA and CTA imaging can obviate the need for duplex carotid Doppler ultrasonography in the evaluation of transient monocular vision loss or amaurosis fugax. Therefore, when asked by emergency room physicians about the best imaging choi   patients with transient ischemic attacks, I often recommend a CTA, which can provide critical information about surgically amenable carotid lesion and can be readily obtained with the baseline CT scan.

Summary

* The choice of best imaging modality in the evaluation of neuro-ophthalmic problems requires recognizing the urgency of the clinical problem, identifying patient-related factors, and localizing the anatomic region of interest.

* The primary goal of the evaluation should be to identify dire diagnoses first, with a view to pursuing more specialized imaging as needed.

* There is much to be gained by discussing cases with the neuroradiologist at your institution. A simple telephone call can go a long way to expediting necessary tests and tailoring the imaging protocol to the region of interest.

* Choosing "which imaging test is best" is part of the art of modern medicine. Experience will be your best teacher.

Bibliography

Beck RW, Trobe JD, Moke PS. High and low-risk profiles for the development of multiple sclerosis within 10-years after optic neuritis: experience of the Optic Neuritis Treatment Trial. *Arch Ophthalmol.* 2003;121:944-949.

Bowen B. MR angiography versus CT angiography in the evaluation of neurovascular disease. *Radiology.* 2007;245:357-361.

Jacobs DA, Galetta SL. Neuro-ophthalmology for neuro-radiologists. *Am J Neuroradiol.* 2007;28:3-8.

Levin LA, Arnold AC. *Neuro-ophthalmology: The Practical Guide.* New York, NY: Thieme Medical Publishers Inc; 2005.

Rodallec MH, Krainik A, Feydy A, et al. Cerebral venous thrombosis and multi-detector CT angiography: tips and tricks. *Radiographics.* 2006;26(Suppl 1):S5-S18.

HOW SHOULD I EVALUATE AND MANAGE SUSPECTED OPTIC NEURITIS?

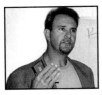

Eric Eggenberger, DO, MSEpi

A 25-year-old woman reports sudden loss of vision OD, pain with eye movement, a right relative afferent pupillary defect, and a normal fundus examination. Right optic neuritis is suspected. What would you recommend for a work-up?

The first step is to firmly establish the diagnosis; you have done most of the clinical work already in that you mention the existence of an afferent pupillary defect and normal fundus. I would certainly want to know the visual acuity, color vision, and visual field for follow-up purposes, but everything you have mentioned thus far points to a retrobulbar optic neuropathy. Together with the history, I agree with you that this is quite consistent with retrobulbar optic neuritis. In particular, periorbital pain is very common (92% in the Optic Neuritis Treatment Trial [ONTT]), and a history of pain with eye movements is often elicited. Despite the fact that this sounds archetypal for retrobulbar optic neuritis, it is worth keeping in mind the possibility of other retrobulbar optic neuropathies if the subsequent clinical course mandates. Nevertheless, we do not order routine labs as part of the initial work-up in such patients.

Working on your diagnosis of retrobulbar optic neuritis, management requires magnetic resonance imaging (MRI), then we need to make an acute therapeutic decision (the use of steroids) followed by a chronic therapeutic decision (consideration of multiple sclerosis [MS] immunomodulatory therapy). I typically order an MRI of brain and orbits with and without contrast (Figures 4-1 and 4-2); the orbital portion helps rule out structural mimics and assists in confirmation (the optic nerve typically enhances if the scan is obtained within the first 3 to 4 weeks). You should be aware that gadolinium-based contrast agents used in MRI may be associated with a progressive fibrosing disease

Figure 4-1. Axial fluid-attenuation inversion recovery (FLAIR) MR study shows periventricular multifocal hyperintense white matter lesions consistent with demyelination.

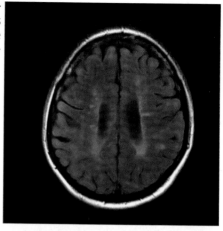

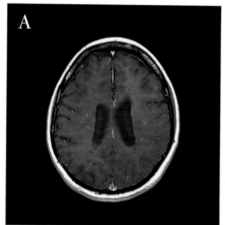
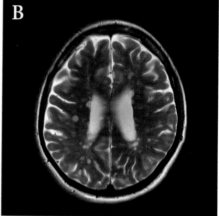

Figure 4-2. (A) Axial T1-weighted MRI post-gadolinium demonstrates enhancing white matter lesions bilaterally. (B) Axial T2-weighted MRI shows periventricular multifocal hyperintense white matter lesions consistent with demyelination.

(nephrogenic systemic fibrosis) in patients with renal failure; additional contraindications to gadolinium contrast include known allergy to the agent or pregnancy. In my opinion, a lumbar puncture is not necessary in the majority of typical optic neuritis cases, although the presence of unique spinal fluid oligoclonal bands may be an independent risk factor for the development of MS, especially if the initial MRI is normal.

The ONTT and its follow-up study, the Longitudinal Optic Neuritis Study (LONS), provide the evidence base for the prognosis of optic neuritis and the use of steroids, and provide data pertaining to the risk of subsequent MS development. The ONTT-randomized patients with acute optic neuritis (<8 days duration) to intravenous (IV) methylprednisolone (250 mg every 6 hours for 3 days followed by a prednisone taper), oral prednisone (1 mg/kg), or placebo. Regardless of treatment group, the prognosis for visual recovery after optic neuritis is generally quite good, with 95% of patients achieving Snellen acuity of 20/40 or better at 12 months; however, the oral prednisone in 1 mg/kg dose in the ONTT was associated with twice the risk of recurrent optic neuritis and is therefore contraindicated. Accordingly, our therapeutic decision involves high-dose methylprednisolone or no steroid therapy. High-dose steroids in the ONTT were associated with a more rapid recovery of visual function, may provide partial protection against the development of MS over the subsequent 2 to 3 years only, and often resolve pain issues rapidly. The potential side effects of steroids are well known and include hyperglycemia, gastrointestinal symptoms, mood alteration (including rare psychosis), insomnia, and the infrequent occurrence of avascular necrosis. Keeping in mind that high-dose steroids merely alter the rate of recovery (not the ultimate extent of recovery), I typically will discuss the risk, benefits, side effects, and alternatives with each patient in light of his or her unique medical history and individual preferences. I tend to offer high-dose methylprednisolone (1 g IV every day for 3 days followed by oral prednisone 1 mg/kg every day for 11 days followed by a 4-day taper) to most patients unless there is a contraindication or patient preference dictates otherwise.

Optic neuritis has a well-known association with MS and is a common first symptom of the disease. The brain portion of the MRI is essential to stratify this patient's risk of subsequent MS and is a key factor in the chronic therapeutic decision we need to make regarding immunomodulatory therapy. The LONS demonstrated that a normal MRI is associated with a 5-year MS risk of 16%, while an abnormal MRI (at least 3 T2 hyperintensities typical of demyelination) corresponds to a 5-year MS risk of 51% (see Figures 4-1 and 4-2). At 10 years, a normal MRI is associated with an MS risk of 22%, while any T2 lesion corresponds to an MS risk of 56%. At 15 years, a normal MRI is associated with an MS risk of 25%, while any T2 abnormality translates to an MS risk of 72%. A normal MRI in combination with certain clinical characteristics also defines a very low MS risk cohort; anterior optic neuritis (ie, papillitis) in a male with a normal MRI is associated with a very low MS risk (only 4% at 15 years). Additionally, with a normal MRI, severe disc edema, disc hemorrhage, painless onset, the presence of a macular star figure, or no light perception visual acuity at onset are features that define a cohort that did not convert to MS even after 15 year follow up.

Trials using interferon beta-1a, interferon beta-1b, or glatiramer acetate in clinically isolated syndrome patients at high risk for MS development have all reported significantly delayed disease progression when these agents are given early (CHAMPS, BENEFIT, and PreCISe trials). The CHAMPS trial randomized patients after a first demyelinating event typical of MS and an MRI with at least 2 T2 lesions to either weekly interferon beta-1a IM or placebo, and approximately 50% of the subjects entered the trial with optic neuritis as their initial demyelinating event. Subjects randomized to interferon beta-1a had a significantly lower conversion rate (42% decreased) to MS compared to subjects on placebo. Very similar findings have since been shown for interferon beta-1b SC qod, and glatiramer acetate.

Summary

* A patient presenting with optic neuritis requires an evaluation that includes clinical history and exam; a targeted MRI scan; and discussion concerning the risk, benefits, side effects, and alternative regarding a treatment course with high-dose steroids.

* In appropriate patients with high-MS risk MRI findings, referral to an MS expert or a similar discussion concerning institution of anti-MS immunomodulatory therapy such as interferons is important for long-term neurologic health.

Bibliography

CHAMPS Study Group. Interferonβ-1a for optic neuritis patients at high risk for multiple sclerosis. *Am J Ophthalmol.* 2001;132:463-471.

Jacobs LD, Beck RW, Simon JH, et al (CHAMPS Study Group). Intramuscular interferon beta-1a therapy initiated during a first demyelinating event in multiple sclerosis. *N Engl J Med.* 2000;343:898-904.

Kaufman DI, Trobe JD, Eggenberger ER, Whitaker JN. Practice parameters: the role of corticosteroids in the management of acute monosymptomatic optic neuritis. *Neurology.* 2000;54:2039-2044.

Optic Neuritis Study Group. The 5-year risk of MS after optic neuritis: experience of the Optic Neuritis Treatment Trial. *Neurology.* 1997;49:1404-1413.

Optic Neuritis Study Group. The clinical profile of acute optic neuritis: experience of the Optic Neuritis Treatment Trial. *Arch Ophthalmol.* 1991;109:1673-1678.

QUESTION 5

WHAT IS THE EVALUATION OF OPTIC NEURITIS?

Steven L. Galetta, MD
(co-authored with Melissa W. Ko, MD)

The patient is a 25-year-old woman with optic neuritis. What are the best treatment options for optic neuritis? Could you tell me how, when, and why should treatment be given for optic neuritis?

The diagnosis of optic neuritis is primarily established by clinical history and examination findings. The first question to be addressed is whether or not the clinical features of the optic neuritis are typical or atypical. In typical optic neuritis, patients describe loss of vision over 7 to 10 days, pain especially with eye movements, and some recovery of vision within 30 days of onset. For these patients, brain magnetic resonance imaging (MRI) should be included in the work-up (T2-weighted, fluid attenuation inversion recovery [FLAIR], T1-weighted gadolinium-enhanced images), primarily for the purpose of prognostication regarding the future risk of multiple sclerosis (MS). Those patients with optic neuritis and white matter abnormalities have the greatest risk of developing MS. At 5 years, 51% of patients with 3 or more white matter lesions that were greater than 3 mm, ovoid, and in the periventricular white matter developed MS in the Optic Neuritis Treatment Trial (ONTT). For those with a normal brain MRI, only 16% developed MS within the first 5 years. Ten years following the initial optic neuritis event, 56% of patients with 1 or more white matter lesions on the baseline brain MRI developed MS. This is in contrast to 22% of patients with a normal baseline MRI who developed MS. At 15 years, 72% of patients with white matter lesions on a brain MRI developed MS while 25% of patients with a normal baseline MRI developed MS.

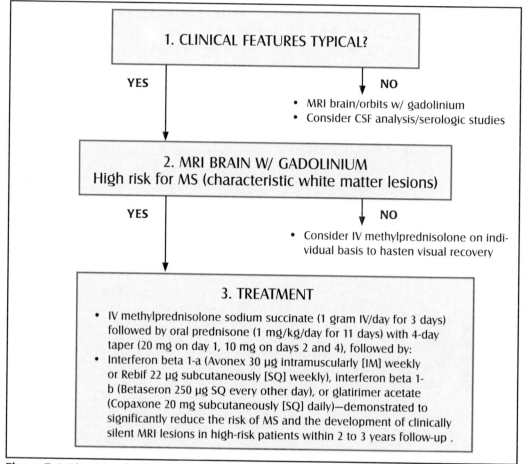

Figure 5-1. Algorithm for the diagnosis and management of the clinically isolated syndrome.

Atypical optic neuritis (ie, infectious, other inflammatory, infiltrative) may require different treatments than idiopathic or demyelinating optic neuritis. Some atypical features for you to consider at presentation include retinal exudates, retinal hemorrhages, severe optic disc edema, no light perception vision, and the absence of pain. When these atypical features are present, in addition to a MRI brain/orbits, I would recommend further diagnostic considerations, including antinuclear antibody test (ANA), fluorescent treponemal antibody absorption (FTA-ABS), angiotensin-converting enzyme (ACE) level, Lyme titer, chest x-ray, and lumbar puncture to look for other causes of optic neuropathy (Figure 5-1). Optical coherence tomography (OCT) and electrophysiological (electroretinogram [ERG], visual evoked response [VER]) studies may be helpful in select cases where the distinction of a retinal condition from an optic nerve process is difficult. The results of these tests might alter your treatment decisions.

In regard to your questions, let me deal first with, "What is the treatment for optic neuritis and how and when should treatment be given?" The ONTT, the largest and most comprehensive study of the optic neuritis patient population to date, has provided important data about the clinical presentation and course of acute demyelinating optic neuritis. This trial, which followed an initial cohort of 457 patients, had the primary objective of determining the effect of intravenous (IV) and oral corticosteroid therapy on visual outcomes in acute demyelinating optic neuritis. Patients were randomized to 1 of 3 treatment groups: 1) oral prednisone (1 mg/kg/day for 14 days with 4-day taper), 2) IV methylprednisolone sodium succinate (250 mg every 6 hours for 3 days followed by oral prednisone [1 mg/kg/day] for 11 days with 4-day taper), or 3) oral placebo.

Patients treated with IV methylprednisolone experienced faster recovery of visual function, particularly in the first 15 days after onset of visual loss, than did patients in the oral prednisone and placebo groups. However, these differences decreased over time until at 1-year follow-up, there were no significant differences in visual function between the treatment groups. Meta-analysis of 12 randomized clinical trials of steroid treatment in MS and optic neuritis showed that corticosteroids improved short-term visual recovery, but there was no statistical benefit in long-term outcomes.

Oral corticosteroids in conventional doses of 60 mg/day should not be used because there was an associated increased risk of optic neuritis recurrence (41%) at 5 years compared to those who received IV methylprednisolone or placebo (25% in both groups). At 10 years from the initial optic neuritis event, the data continued to show that recurrence risk of optic neuritis was still higher in the oral prednisone (44%) versus the IV group (29%). There was no statistical difference in recurrence of optic neuritis between oral prednisone and the placebo group. Therefore, the decision to use corticosteroids for visual recovery alone needs to be individualized and IV steroids are the recommended regimen. If oral corticosteroids need to be used (insurance issues, access problems, etc) in a patient with acute optic neuritis, we would recommend a high-dose oral regimen of 1000 mg methylprednisolone for 3 days, but this treatment regimen has not been adequately studied in a large cohort of patients with optic neuritis. For patients with optic neuritis and 2 or more high-signal abnormalities on baseline brain MRI, IV corticosteroids may delay MS onset, but the effect is short-lived and by 3 years treated versus untreated groups had a similar risk of developing MS. Nonetheless, it is common practice to administer high-dose IV corticosteroids to optic neuritis patients at high risk for MS irrespective of the extent of their visual impairment.

There have been several important studies involving treatment with interferon beta in patients experiencing a first clinical event suggestive of MS. The first of these trials, CHAMPS, enrolled patients with a recent history (within 14 days) of a demyelinating event, a large subset of which were patients with optic neuritis. These patients also had brain MRI findings consistent with high risk for clinically definite MS as established by the ONTT. Patients randomized to the treatment group received weekly intramuscular injections of 30 µg interferon beta-1a (Avonex [Biogen, Cambridge, MA]). Patients who received interferon beta-1a had a 44% reduction in the 3-year risk of developing clinical definite MS (CDMS) compared to placebo. In addition, these patients showed a reduced rate of accumulation of new but clinically silent lesions on brain MRI.

A similar trial by the Early Treatment of MS (ETOMS) Study Group also yielded results that demonstrated a benefit for interferon beta-1a treatment following a first clinical demyelinating event such as optic neuritis. Patients with both neurologic and radiologic evidence of a first demyelinating event were randomized to weekly injections of subcutaneous interferon beta-1a 22 µg (Rebif [Serono Pharmaceutical, Rockland, MA]) or placebo within 3 months of symptoms and were monitored over a 2-year period. Comparable to the findings of the previous interferon beta-1a trials, ETOMS found a lower risk of developing clinically definite MS (34% versus 45%, p=0.047), as well as a lower annual relapse rate (0.33 versus 0.43, p=0.045) in the treatment group compared to placebo. Disease activity, as measured by lesion burden on MRI, was also significantly lower. In a related study of the same cohort, patients receiving interferon beta-1a demonstrated a reduced rate of brain volume loss over 2 years, suggesting that early treatment with interferon beta-1a may have the additional benefit of slowing the progressive loss of brain parenchyma that is frequently seen in patients with MS. Glatirimer acetate (Copaxone, Teva Pharmaceutical, Israel) has also shown benefit in delaying the onset of clinically definite MS in a monofocal cohort of clinically isolated syndrome patients.

More recent trials have focused on interferon beta-1b (Betaseron [Bayer Healthcare Pharmaceutical, Montville, NJ]), also an established treatment for relapsing remitting MS. The BENEFIT Study, a randomized, placebo-controlled phase III trial, demonstrated that treatment with interferon beta-1b delayed the development of clinically definite MS as defined by the Poser criteria (CDMS = second clinical demyelinating event), and also by the more recently established McDonald criteria, which incorporate MRI findings of dissemination of lesions in time and space. BENEFIT-enrolled patients with clinical evidence of a first demyelinating event and at least 2 clinically silent lesions on MRI suggestive of MS. The treatment group received interferon beta-1b 250 µg administered every other day by subcutaneous injection. At 2 years follow-up, the probability of developing clinically definite MS was 28% in the treatment group compared to 45% in the placebo group. Risk for developing MS as defined by the McDonald criteria was reduced from 85% to 69%. Secondary efficacy variables, which reflect the burden of inflammatory lesions on MRI scan, also demonstrated positive treatment effects. This study also demonstrated a reduction of disability progression in the immediately treated group compared to those patients who received delayed interferon therapy.

With the advent of long-term therapy options, it is reasonable to consider whether it is necessary or beneficial to begin indefinite therapy for a chronic disease with a variable natural course. Many physicians argue that we cannot consistently identify such patients and that we may risk long-term, irreversible disability by delaying treatment. Some physicians advocate an initial observation period to better determine the patient's disease progression before initiating therapy. They argue that many patients could avoid long-term therapy—and the financial expense and adverse effects that accompany it—without affecting the patient's prognosis. Until we can reliably determine which patients can safely defer treatment, we recommend offering long-term immunomodulatory therapy to all patients with a first demyelinating event whose MRI suggests high risk for MS.

Summary

* The use of corticosteroids must be individualized in the patient with optic neuritis. If there are white matter lesions suspicious for demyelination, use of IV corticosteroids is suggested. IV corticosteroids can hasten visual recovery and delay MS onset, but the effect is short lived and by 3 years treated versus placebo groups had a similar risk of developing MS.

* There is no role for oral corticosteroids at conventional doses because studies have demonstrated an increased risk of optic neuritis recurrence.

∗ MRI brain with contrast is an important part of the evaluation to assess future MS risk.

∗ Initiation of interferon therapy is recommended in those optic neuritis patients with high-signal white matter lesions typical of demyelination on brain MRI. Multiple trials have demonstrated that interferon therapy reduces the risk of developing CDMS. In addition, some trials showed that immediate treatment following the initial demyelinating event reduced both the probability of developing CDMS and the development of clinically silent MRI lesions in high-risk patients several years following the event.

WHAT IS NEURORETINITIS?

Rod Foroozan, MD

The patient is an 18-year-old man with visual loss due to optic disc edema and a macular star figure OD. The left eye is normal. "Neuroretinitis" is suspected. What is the appropriate evaluation and treatment for this condition?

It sounds like your patient does have "neuroretinitis." This is a term used to describe optic disc edema in combination with lipid exudate within the macula and fovea, typically in the configuration of a macular star (Figure 6-1). Although more than one type of optic neuropathy (including anterior ischemic optic neuropathy, hypertensive retinopathy, and papilledema) can cause optic disc edema with exudate in the configuration of a macular star, when I use the term *neuroretinitis* I am implying an inflammatory cause for the optic neuropathy. I find that one of the most frequently found, and often overlooked, signs in patients with neuroretinitis is the presence of inflammatory cells within the vitreous, which are nearly uniformly present and help suggest that the problem is from inflammation. Neuroretinitis is most commonly unilateral but inflammatory signs, such as foci of retinitis, may be bilateral and the optic disc edema can uncommonly be bilateral. The optic disc edema precedes the development of the macular exudate.

Visual dysfunction from neuroretinitis is quite variable and occurs from a combination of retinopathy and optic neuropathy, and it may be difficult to determine which problem is more severe. The presence of a relative afferent pupillary defect and dense visual field defects suggest an optic neuropathy. Optical coherence tomography (OCT) can be helpful to determine and follow the degree of maculopathy (Figure 6-2).

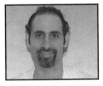

Figure 6-1. Optic disc edema with macular star in the right eye of a patient with cat-scratch disease. There is an adjacent yellow deep retinal- or choroidal-based lesion inferotemporal to the optic disc.

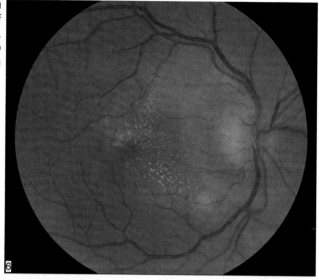

Figure 6-2. OCT of the right eye of the patient in Figure 6-1 shows subretinal fluid in the area of the fovea.

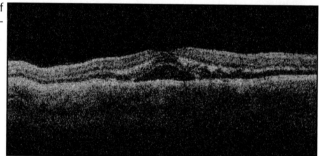

The causes of neuroretinitis are varied and include 2 broad categories: 1) sterile inflammation and 2) infection (Table 6-1). Traditionally, multiple sclerosis has not been associated with neuroretinitis, but demyelinating optic neuritis can be a cause, although in that case cells in the vitreous are unexpected. Despite the entities listed in Table 6-1, and several more exhaustive ones, a number of patients (perhaps 50%) with neuroretinitis will have no specific cause identified. I would estimate that about 25% to 50% of the patients I see with neuroretinitis have cat-scratch disease as the underlying cause. These patients often have waxing and waning fever that precedes the onset of visual loss. The visual symptoms often begin several weeks after exposure to the infected cat (in nearly all the patients I have seen it has been from kittens and not adult cats, although direct infection from fleas may also play a role). In association with the optic disc edema there are often focal areas of retinitis (Figure 6-3) that may resemble cotton wool spots but will show leakage on fluorescein angiography or deeper yellow/white lesions that are subretinal or choroidal based (see Figure 6-1). Fluorescein angiography may also show leakage and staining of the optic disc. It is leakage of the vessels of the optic disc that is thought to contribute to the macular exudate. There may be retinal hemorrhages and retinal vasculitis with artery or vein occlusions.

An important component in the evaluation of patients with neuroretinitis is a review of systems for inflammatory conditions. I would start by asking about systemic

Table 6-1

Possible Causes of Neuroretinitis

Sterile Inflammation	Infection	Infectious Organism
Demyelinating optic neuritis (rare)		
Sarcoidosis		
Vasculitis		
	Viruses	Epstein-Barr virus
		Hepatitis B
	Bacteria	*Bartonella henselae* (common)
		Rickettsial disease
		Mycobacterium tuberculosis
	Spirochetes	*Treponema pallidum*
		Borrelia burgdorferi
	Protozoa	*Toxoplasma gondii*

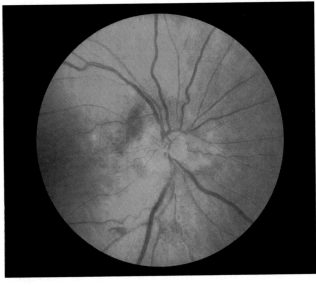

Figure 6-3. There is a white focus of retinitis just between the fovea and optic disc in the right eye of a patient with optic disc edema from cat-scratch disease.

symptoms and conditions such as fever and night sweats, pulmonary disease, joint swelling, skin rash, sexually transmitted disease, travel (eg, to areas endemic for Lyme disease or Rocky Mountain spotted fever), exposure to animals (including kittens), occupational history (animal handler), and dietary history (ingestion of uncooked meat).

If the history and findings are classic for cat-scratch disease, then the only ancillary test I would suggest is *Bartonella henselae* titers. In the absence of findings suggestive of one of the specific conditions in Table 6-1, I typically start by ordering the following blood tests: complete blood count, erythrocyte sedimentation rate, Lyme titer, rapid plasma reagin (RPR), fluorescent treponemal antibody (FTA-ABS), and serum angiotensin-converting enzyme (ACE). Otherwise I order additional testing on a patient-by-patient basis (eg, a chest x-ray and skin testing in a patient suspected of having tuberculosis, *Toxoplasma gondii* titers in a patient with chorioretinal infiltrates and an adjacent scar, or c-antineutrophilic cytoplasmic antibody [ANCA] and p-ANCA in a patient suspected of having vasculitis). Although a number of viruses have been reported to cause neuroretinitis, in the absence of systemic symptoms suggestive of a particular viral syndrome I typically do not order viral titers because most of these conditions are self-limited and without a specific treatment.

In patients without a specific cause for the neuroretinitis, I typically order an MRI of the brain and orbits with fat suppression and contrast, unless the optic disc edema has already subsided (often with an improvement in visual function). Many of the causes of neuroretinitis, including cat-scratch disease, may be associated with other central nervous system findings, including meningeal enhancement or parenchymal disease.

I typically do not suggest a lumbar puncture for patients with isolated unilateral neuroretinitis, but reserve it for patients with bilateral optic disc edema or those with neuroretinitis and other findings suggestive of neurologic dysfunction. Likewise, I do not suggest consultation with a neurologist unless other concurrent neurologic dysfunction is present or there are unexpected neuroimaging findings. Consultation with an infectious disease specialist may be helpful for those with neuroretinitis and other neurologic dysfunction or systemic symptoms, especially as new agents are developed to treat the infectious causes.

Most patients with neuroretinitis show spontaneous improvement in visual function, especially those who have more profound macular edema, within weeks to months of the onset of visual loss. In my experience those patients with more severe optic neuropathy have a worse prognosis than those with more severe maculopathy. As the macular star improves, there are commonly some changes in the foveal retinal pigmental epithelium that tend to be permanent. Spontaneous improvement is one factor that has made the determination of a treatment benefit controversial. Although most commonly it occurs as a single event, some patients may have recurrent neuroretinitis with poor visual outcomes.

There is some evidence that treatment with antibiotics (a number of different agents have been found to be effective) is helpful for the systemic findings (including lymph node enlargement) in cat-scratch disease. However, there is no proof that treatment is helpful for improving neuroretinitis. My preference is to treat with azithromycin for 2 weeks, and I have seen patients with optic disc edema but without macular pathology who have been treated with antibiotics and avoided the development of an exudative maculopathy. Thus my own bias is that antibiotics are helpful, even for the ocular findings in cat-scratch disease. For the other specific causes of neuroretinitis, treatment of the specific systemic condition is important but its effects on the ocular findings are less certain. Some clinicians have suggested that corticosteroids be used concurrently with antibiotics. I typically do not use them unless there is evidence of progressive visual loss or I am more concerned about a sterile cause of inflammation such as sarcoidosis. The benefit of additional treatment measures such as intravitreal corticosteroid injections or periocular injections is without much evidence but can be considered in a patient-by-patient basis.

Summary

* Neuroretinitis is an inflammatory optic neuropathy characterized by optic disc edema and lipid within the fovea in a macular star pattern.
* Neuroretinitis is often associated with cells in the vitreous.
* Sterile inflammation and infection are the two broad types of disorders which cause neuroretinitis.
* Cat scratch disease is the single most common cause of neuroretinitis.
* Neuroretinitis generally has a good prognosis with spontaneous improvement, which has made assessment of treatment difficult.

Bibliography

Cunningham ET, Koehler JE. Ocular bartonellosis. *Am J Ophthalmol*. 2000;130:340-349.
Ray S, Gragoudas E. Neuroretinitis. *Int Ophthalmol Clin*. 2001;41:83-102.

HOW DO YOU EVALUATE NON-ARTERITIC ANTERIOR ISCHEMIC OPTIC NEUROPATHY?

M. Tariq Bhatti, MD

The patient is a 45-year-old man with acute onset visual loss OD. He has a right relative afferent papillary defect (RAPD) and a swollen optic nerve OD. The left eye is normal. He has some pain but no pain with eye movement. Can you tell me how you would go about making the diagnosis of non-arteritic anterior ischemic optic neuropathy versus optic neuritis or another optic neuropathy?

A middle-aged gentleman with a right optic neuropathy associated with pain, which I assume is in the region of the right eye, and a swollen optic nerve, is a tough case. At 45 years of age, the 2 most common causes of a swollen optic nerve are non-arteritic anterior ischemic optic neuropathy (NAION) and optic neuritis (ON). However, it should be noted that the differential diagnosis of a swollen optic nerve is extensive and includes other inflammatory, vascular, orbital, toxic/metabolic, hereditary, infiltrative, and compressive causes. If we are to assume this is NAION, the diagnosis is based on the history, clinical examination, and disease course. In other words, NAION is a clinical diagnosis. If laboratory evaluation and neuroimaging are performed, it is often done to exclude other possibilities such as ON and the multitude of vascular, infectious, neoplastic, and inflammatory optic neuropathies.

In this patient, a key piece of information that is very helpful in the diagnosis is the fact that he has pain but not with eye movements. This is important because approximately 90% of patients with ON will have eye pain exacerbated by eye movements compared to only 10% of patients with NAION who note mild eye pain without eye movements. If we were dealing with someone over the age of 50 years, it would be critical to ascertain a

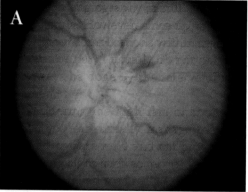 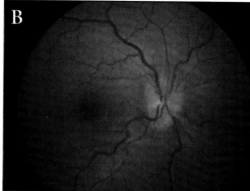

Figure 7-1. (A) Diffusely swollen and hyperemic optic nerve due to NAION. (B) Mild optic nerve swelling in the setting of optic neuritis.

Figure 7-2. Inferior altitudinal visual field defect in a left eye of a patient suffering from NAION.

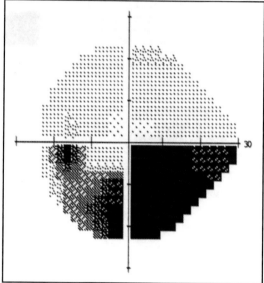

history of headaches, scalp tenderness, jaw claudication, weight loss, or neck pain for the possibility of arteritic anterior ischemic optic neuropathy due to temporal arteritis.

If the rest of the ocular examination is normal including no evidence of intraocular inflammation, as is the case with NAION, then I would concentrate on the significance of the optic nerve swelling. Typically with NAION the optic nerve is either diffusely or segmentally swollen with pallor, hemorrhages, and arteriolar attenuation (Figure 7-1A). This is in contrast to the optic nerve swelling seen with ON, which is often mild, diffuse, and without hemorrhages or arteriolar attenuation (Figure 7-1B). The configuration of the fellow optic nerve should also be noted in any patient suspected of NAION. A small cup-to-disc ratio is present and is termed *the disc at risk* in the vast majority of cases. Visual field testing typically shows an inferior altitudinal defect in NAION (Figure 7-2), but any optic nerve-related visual field loss may occur.

The vision remains relatively stable in most patients with NAION. However, I caution patients that they may continue to lose vision while the optic nerve is swollen.

Progressive visual loss can occur over 6 to 8 weeks in approximately one-third of patients. Forty percent of patients may show spontaneous visual improvement of 3 lines of vision or more 6 months from the onset of the visual loss. There are a few recommendations I would make regarding your patient's diagnostic work-up. Although my suspicion is high that he has NAION given the pain and the relatively young age, a magnetic resonance imaging (MRI) of the brain and orbits with contrast could be offered to evaluate for the possibility of demyelinating disease.

I do not routinely order an echocardiogram or carotid doppler because embolic, cardiac, or aortic arch disease is rarely a cause of NAION, especially if there is no evidence of retinal emboli on the clinical examination. This patient is too young for temporal arteritis, but a sedimentation rate, C-reactive protein, and a complete blood count could be performed in a case of an older person.

Although the exact pathogenesis of NAION is not known, it is thought to be a vasculopathy of the paraoptic branches of the posterior ciliary arteries that feed the retrolaminar portion of the optic nerve head. A variety of risk factors have been associated with NAION, including diabetes mellitus, arterial hypertension, nocturnal hypotension, hyperlipidemia, optic disc morphology ("disc at risk"), medications (ie, amiodarone, sildenafil citrate), migraine, and optic nerve drusen. If the patient does not have the "big three" (ie, diabetes mellitus, arterial hypertension, and hyperlipidemia), I would recommend a complete physical examination and blood work-up by the primary physician or internist. There is some controversy whether patients with NAION are truly at an increased risk of cerebrovascular accidents or ischemic cardiac disease compared to the general population. If the patient has diabetes mellitus, arterial hypertension, hyperlipidemia, or history of smoking cigarettes, then risk modification is strongly encouraged.

Patients with NAION in one eye should be counseled that there is an approximately 15% chance of fellow eye involvement in the next 5 years. Although controversial, you could start daily aspirin therapy if there is no contraindication. Unfortunately, there is no proven therapy for the treatment of NAION. Optic nerve sheath fenestration was found to be ineffective and in some cases harmful. A variety of medications including topical brimonidine, oral corticosteroids, anticoagulants, thrombolytic agents, levodopa, and diphenylhydantoin, and recently intravitreal bevacizumab (Avastin [Genentech, San Francisco, CA]) have all been reported but unproven therapies in NAION.

Patients should be monitored until the optic nerve swelling resolves, which usually occurs within 4 to 6 weeks. Either diffuse or segmental optic nerve pallor becomes evident at this time and is associated with a fixed visual field defect. It is very rare for a second ischemic event to occur in an eye with a previous attack of NAION, but if this happens, I would consider performing a complete hypercoagulable and inflammatory work-up. I also remind patients who have suffered NAION in one eye on the nearly 3.5-fold increased risk of NAION with cataract surgery in the fellow eye.

Summary

* NAION is a clinical diagnosis.
* Evaluation and management of vasculopathic risk factors is recommended.
* Optic nerve decompression is not recommended for NAION.

✳ There are no proven treatments for NAION.

Bibliography

Arnold AC. Pathogenesis of nonarteritic anterior ischemic optic neuropathy. *J Neuroophthalmol.* 2003;23:157-163.

Bennett JL, Thomas S, Olson JL, Mandava N. Treatment of nonarteritic anterior ischemic optic neuropathy with intravitreal bevacizumab. *J Neuroophthalmol.* 2007;27:238-240.

Newman NJ, Scherer R, Langenberg P, et al. The fellow eye in NAION: report from the ischemic optic neuropathy decompression trial follow-up study. *Am J Ophthalmol.* 2002;134:317-328.

The Ischemic Optic Neuropathy Decompression Trial Research Group. Optic nerve decompression surgery for nonarteritic anterior ischemic optic neuropathy (NAION) is not effective and may be harmful. *JAMA.* 1995;273:625-632.

Warner JE, Lessell S, Rizzo JF 3rd, Newman NJ. Does optic disc appearance distinguish ischemic optic neuropathy from optic neuritis? *Arch Ophthalmol.* 1997;115:1408-1410.

How Do You Differentiate Arteritic Anterior Ischemic Optic Neuropathy From Non-Arteritic?

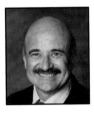

Alfredo A. Sadun, MD, PhD

A 76-year-old woman experienced acute visual loss OD, a right relative afferent pupillary defect (RAPD), and a pale, swollen optic nerve OD. There is an adjacent cilioretinal artery occlusion as well. Arteritic (giant cell arteritis) anterior ischemic optic neuropathy (AION) is suspected. Can you tell me how you want to proceed?

As in most problems in neuro-ophthalmology, the history provides the most useful and important information. In your patient's case, we are dealing with a 76-year-old woman who presents with a sudden loss of vision. The combination of age and suddenness automatically should elicit suspicion for giant cell arteritis. This in turn should bring about a series of questions looking for constitutional and systemic signs and symptoms of the disease. I always ask about headaches, jaw claudication, scalp tenderness, myalgias, fever, fatigue, appetite, and weight loss. It is important for you to ask about jaw claudication correctly as this might be the most specific sign for giant cell arteritis (also called temporal arteritis). We are not talking about chronic, mandibular pain or pain and clicking upon opening the jaw. Rather, we are talking about ischemic claudication-type aching that is associated with the chewing of firm food. Indeed, most patients with this symptom admit to changing their dietary habits to avoid certain foods such as meat and crusty breads.

It is also very important to ask this woman whether preceding her abrupt loss of vision there were episodes of transient obscurations of vision that may have lasted minutes. These transient episodes of darkening, or constriction of the visual field, are highly suggestive for arteritic AION.

Figure 8-1. Fundus photograph showing pale and swollen optic disc with adjacent cilioretinal artery occlusion suggestive of giant cell arteritis.

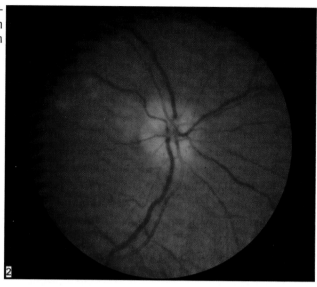

A comprehensive neuro-ophthalmological examination is required. Additionally, it is particularly useful to examine and palpate the temporal arteries. Are they tender? Are they nodular? Is the pulse obliterated? Any affirmative answer further raises the index of suspicion for giant cell arteritis. In this case, fundus examination reflected a pale swollen optic nerve. Patients with posterior optic neuropathy (PION) would initially have no fundus findings, though later, as in all optic neuropathies, optic atrophy would ensue. PION may be related to shock-like conditions (often perioperative) or be due to giant cell arteritis. In this case, however, with optic disc edema we are talking about AION. Often there are peripapillary hemorrhages in addition to the swollen optic nerve. It may be impossible to distinguish between the arteritic and non-arteritic forms of AION on funduscopy alone. However, evidence of "pallid edema" (Figure 8-1) as opposed to hyperemia points toward the diagnosis of arteritic AION. Funduscopy can also provide us with information about the optic nerve head configuration in the fellow eye. In non-arteritic AION, one generally sees a very small optic cup.

The abrupt onset of visual loss due to an optic neuropathy is often ischemic in nature. Ischemic optic neuropathies may be anterior (with disc edema) or posterior. PION is often associated with significant blood loss leading to anemia and often there is concomitant hypotension. However, it may also be due to giant cell arteritis. Non-arteritic AION is usually a spontaneous event that occurs to patients in a 50- to 80-year age range and has 2 general categories of risk factors: 1) an anatomical predisposition known as "disc at risk" consistent with a very small cup-to-disc ratio and 2) a vasculopathic element (most often diabetes, hypertension, or hyperlipidemia). However, in the elderly (usually persons 70 years of age or older), arteritic anterior ischemic optic neuropathy (AAION means AION secondary to giant cell arteritis) becomes ever more likely. Since patients with giant cell arteritis may have an ischemic optic neuropathy in one eye and then shortly thereafter go blind in the other eye, prompt diagnosis and treatment is extremely important. This is particularly true since there are effective modalities of treatment for giant cell arteritis.

The first thing I would recommend is for you to be suspicious of the disease in every older patient with visual loss. I recommend thinking of giant cell arteritis whenever an elderly patient complains of either visual loss or diplopia (arteritis causes cranial nerve palsies too). Then it is incumbent upon the physician to ask the right questions (see history above). The physical examination is also useful (see above). Fluorescein angiogram may also be useful, as in giant cell arteritis there is a delay in choroidal filling as well as in optic disc filling. If there remains any doubt in the clinician's mind, then 3 blood tests might be useful in confirming the diagnosis. The erythrocyte sedimentation rate (ESR) is easily available and often can be obtained within 1 to 2 hours. The old rule of thumb (a guideline and not always true) is that if the ESR is higher than the patient's age plus 10 and divided by 2 (for women) or the patient's age plus 5 and divided by 2 (for men), then the ESR should be regarded as suspicious for giant cell arteritis. So, in the example above, a 76-year-old woman would bring us concern if her ESR was higher than 43 (76 plus 10 divided by 2). Of course, a high ESR is very nonspecific. Hence, it is useful to get in addition a measure of serum C-reactive protein (CRP). I also get a complete blood count (CBC) since many patients with giant cell arteritis suffer from chronic anemia and thrombocytosis. Hayreh et al have published sensitivities and specificities higher than 95% when using both ESR and CRP to rule out giant cell arteritis in cases of AION.

Confirmation of the diagnosis of giant cell arteritis may be made by a biopsy of the superficial temporal artery. Histopathological confirmation comes primarily from the identification of macrophages and giant cells and extensive disruption of the internal limiting elastica. These changes will persist for at least 2 or 3 weeks after the initiation of corticosteroid treatment (and sometimes much longer) and hence patients should be put on corticosteroid treatment prior to the biopsy. The temporal artery biopsy has a sensitivity and specificity of approximately 97%.

The most important thing is to treat while you are waiting. I generally put a patient, in whom I have a significant degree of suspicion of giant cell arteritis, on 60 to 80 mg of prednisone a day. Additionally, many neuro-ophthalmologists choose to admit the patient for high-dose intravenous (IV) steroids (g a day of methylprednisolone) for 2 or 3 days and possibly heparin therapy as well. Often the patients are maintained on aspirin thereafter. The clinician is reminded that the natural history of giant cell arteritis involves very long-term changes. Patients may need to be treated for up 2 years or, sometimes, even longer. Usually, I adjust the dosage of prednisone by titration against monthly ESRs. I generally create a target ESR based on the patient's age and other systemic issues (adjusting the ESR up if the patient has arthritis or diabetes, etc). When the ESR drops far below this target, I then slowly adjust the prednisone dose down but I never allow the ESR to go higher than the target that I had previously set. Typically, a patient may begin on prednisone 80 mg a day and be at perhaps 30 mg at 3 months, 20 mg at 6 months, and 10 mg at 1 year. However, every patient is adjusted according to his or her own signs, symptoms, and—most particularly—ESR. Finally, there are many patients who do not tolerate corticosteroids well and these patients may be put on steroid-sparing agents instead. The rheumatologist can help with this. However, I always begin my patients with prednisone first, as these doses can be manipulated more adroitly.

Summary

* Always maintain a high index of suspicion for giant cell arteritis especially in the elderly patient.

* Ask the right questions.

* Get an ESR, CBC, and CRP and have a very low threshold of suspicion.

* Initiate therapy with systemic corticosteroids first and get a temporal artery biopsy second.

Bibliography

Arnold AC. Ischemic optic neuropathy, diabetic papillopathy, and papillophlebitis. In: Yanoff M, Duker J, eds. *Ophthalmology*. St. Louis, MO: Mosby; 2004:1268-1274.

Boyev LR, Miller NR, Green WR. Efficacy of unilateral vs. bilateral temporal artery biopsy's for the diagnosis of giant cell arteritis. *Am J Ophthalmol*. 1999;128:211-215.

Hayreh SS, Podhajsky PA, Raman R, et al. Giant cell arteritis: validity reliability of various diagnostic criteria. *Am J Ophthalmol*. 1997;123:285-296.

Hayreh SS, Podhajsky PA, Zimmerman P. Ocular manifestations of giant cell arteritis. *Am J Ophthalmol*. 1998;125:509-520.

HOW LONG DO YOU HAVE TO TREAT GIANT CELL ARTERITIS?

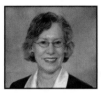

Jacqueline A. Leavitt, MD

The patient is a 70-year-old woman with osteoporosis and a history of falls. Now she has developed new no light perception in the right eye and a pale swollen right optic nerve. A temporal artery biopsy was positive for giant cell arteritis (GCA). In dealing with a patient with biopsy-proven GCA, how long should steroid therapy last?

There is no firm timeline for the long-term treatment of GCA with steroids. In general the treatment of GCA is with oral glucocorticoids and normally starts with a daily dose of 60 to 80 mg. Treatment should be started even before the temporal artery biopsy is done, as long as the biopsy will be done within a week or so. I have found that most patients begin to feel better after steroid therapy within a few days. It has been our experience at the Mayo Clinic that the steroids often can be tapered slowly beginning about 1 month after onset of treatment and then tapering down by about 10 mg/week so that within a few months the patient is on a modest dose (10 to 20 mg/d). Slower tapering of the daily dosage by 1-mg increments and then continuing for a total treatment regimen of 9 to 18 months treats most patients. Some patients, however, can discontinue steroids faster while others might require lifelong low-dose maintenance therapy.

Some people advocate using intravenous (IV) steroids to treat GCA. These authors often start the patients on 1 g of IV methylprednisolone daily. There are only a few reports that have looked at this issue, and there is no strong evidence to support the use of IV steroids over oral steroids.

I use the patient's symptoms and the blood tests (ie, erythrocyte sedimentation rate [ESR], C-reactive protein [CRP]) to determine the rate of the steroid taper. The absence of new or worsening clinical symptoms as well as a normal ESR and CRP generally indicate that continued slow tapering or discontinuation of treatment is possible. If the patient experiences any recurrence of his or her symptoms or develops new ischemic symptoms or a marked elevation of the ESR and/or CRP, then increasing or restarting the steroid therapy is warranted.

Prolonged steroids can be associated with significant side effects (eg, weight gain, glucose intolerance, hypertension, osteoporosis, avascular necrosis, opportunistic infections). Although in other disorders side effects are much less with every-other-day dosing of steroids, this regimen does not provide adequate therapy for GCA and I do not recommend every-other-day therapy in GCA. On the other hand, steroid-sparing agents are sometimes used to alleviate steroid side effects. Unfortunately, there are only 2 studies using methotrexate in place of steroids for treatment of GCA and each study came to a different and opposite conclusion on efficacy. Nevertheless, steroid-sparing regimens including methotrexate may have a role in patients with GCA.

One of the infrequent complications from GCA is aortic aneurysm. Patients with GCA were found to be 17 times more likely to develop an aortic aneurysm and 2.4 times more likely to develop an isolated abdominal aortic aneurysm then the age- and sex-matched controls in an Olmsted County incidence study. Aortic dissection is another complication associated with GCA and these might be additional arguments for maintaining steroid therapy for a longer duration in addition to control of the constitutional symptoms and prevention of further visual loss.

Summary

* GCA typically requires high-dose corticosteroids with a slow taper over months to years.

* IV steroids have not been proven to be more effective than oral steroids but could be considered at presentation in selected patients.

* There are no clinical trials to guide the length of treatment in GCA.

* The patient's clinical course, laboratory testing (eg, ESR, CRP), and the clinician's judgment are the best ways to determine a treatment and tapering plan for the individual patient with GCA.

Bibliography

Chevalet P, Barrier JH, Pottier P, et al. A randomized, multicenter, controlled trial using intravenous pulses of methylprednisolone in the initial treatment of simple forms of giant cell arteritis: a one year follow study of 164 patients. *J Rheumatol.* 2000;27:1484-1491.

Evans JM, O'Fallon WM, Hunder GG. Increased incidence of aortic aneurysm and dissection in giant cell (temporal) arteritis: a population-based study. *Ann Intern Med.* 1975;122:502-507.

Hoffman GS, Cid MC, Hellmann DB, et al. A multicenter, randomized, double-blind, placebo-controlled trial of adjuvant methotrexate treatment for giant cell arteritis. *Arthritis & Rheumatism.* 2002;46:1309-1318.

Jover JA, Hernandez-Garcia C, Morado IC, et al. Treatment of giant-cell arteritis with methotrexate and prednisone: a randomized, double-blind, placebo-controlled trial. *Ann Intern Med.* 2001;134:106-114.

Klein RG, Hunder GG, Stanson AW, Sheps SG. Large artery involvement in giant cell (temporal) arteritis. *Ann Intern Med.* 1975;83:806-812.

WHAT IS THE EVALUATION OF TRAUMATIC OPTIC NEUROPATHY?

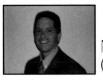

Nicholas J. Volpe, MD
(co-authored with Jennifer K. Hall, MD)

A 20-year-old man struck his right forehead after flipping over his bicycle. He did not lose consciousness and has no other neurologic symptoms. He was seen in the emergency room and discharged and he has been complaining of visual loss OD. He has a right relative afferent pupillary defect (RAPD), but a normal-appearing optic disc OD. The left eye was normal. It is believed he has traumatic optic neuropathy (TON). What imaging if any should be performed? Steroids cannot hurt, right?

Your patient's story and presentation would indeed raise high suspicion for TON. Traumatic injury to the optic nerve can occur through either direct or indirect mechanisms. Direct injury is caused by penetrating trauma, while a blow to the brow or facial eminences can cause indirect injury. Optic nerve avulsion (partial or complete severance of the optic nerve from the globe), can occur via direct on indirect mechanisms. Indirect TON is typically subdivided into optic nerve avulsion and posterior indirect traumatic optic neuropathy. The story above is most consistent with posterior indirect TON. The incidence of TON is highest in young men (as is any trauma), with bicycle and motor vehicle accidents providing the most common setting. Other causes include injuries from falling objects, gunshots, assault, and skateboards. TON can occur after seemingly minor trauma. The incidence is 2% to 5% after facial trauma.

Criteria associated with the diagnosis of posterior indirect TON include decreased acuity and color vision, a visual field defect, a RAPD in unilateral cases, normal-appearing fundus and external exam, and a history of trauma. In most cases, because the injury is to the facial bones, the globe is normal with no evidence of traumatic iritis, hyphema, vitreous hemorrhage, or commotio retinae. The visual field defect can take any form, although altitudinal defects and central scotomas are common. Visual acuity is often 20/400 or worse, however, acuity can range from 20/20 to no light perception. Vision loss from indirect posterior TON is often biphasic, with immediate compromise followed by delayed worsening. Direct TON is diagnosed based on history and clinical or radiologic evidence of penetrating injury. In cases of optic nerve avulsion, a complete or partial ring of hemorrhage can be seen at the optic disc. In general, diagnoses to rule out when considering TON include pre-existing optic neuropathy, retinal compromise secondary to trauma, and functional (nonorganic) vision loss.

I typically recommend that a computed tomography (CT) scan be done as part of the work-up of a suspected TON. Direct coronal cuts (1.5 mm) are desirable if the patient can be positioned safely, but newer CT coronal reconstructions can also be satisfactory. This allows superior evaluation of the optic canal. The canal should be carefully examined for any fractures, and in particular for bony fragments that may be impinging on the nerve. Other findings that might be amenable to surgical treatment include an optic nerve sheath or subperiosteal hematoma or hemorrhage in the orbital apex, sphenoid sinus, or ethmoid sinus. Once a metallic foreign body or other contraindications are ruled out, magnetic resonance imaging (MRI) can be employed to better evaluate soft tissue abnormalities but may not be necessary. CT can also play a role in surgical planning for an optic canal decompression.

In direct TON, a penetrating object causes direct injury to the nerve. Optic nerve avulsion can occur in this manner, or it can occur secondary to indirect trauma in the setting of twisting forces on the globe. Injury from indirect posterior TON most commonly occurs within the optic canal. Following a frontal blow, sudden deceleration of the head with continued forward motion of the globe causes shearing forces along the intracanalicular nerve where it has firm dural attachments. Additionally, it has been demonstrated that anterior-most portion of the canal, the optic foramen, is the major site of transmitted force from frontal blows. While the optic canal is the most common site for injury in the setting of posterior indirect TON, the second most common site is the intracranial optic nerve. Involvement of the chiasm can also be seen.

Immediate vision loss from posterior indirect TON is thought to occur secondary to mechanical shearing of axons as well as contusion necrosis secondary to ischemia from microvasculature compromise. A combination of apoptotic mechanisms, reperfusion injury, and edema is thought to be responsible for delayed vision loss.

Currently, there is no evidence-based standard of care for the treatment of TON. Spontaneous improvement in acuity occurs in many patients. Treatment options have included steroids and/or optic canal decompression. There have been no randomized clinical trials to support either of these modalities, and no clear consensus on the efficacy of these treatments has emerged from multiple retrospective or prospective descriptive studies. Additionally, the National Acute Spinal Cord Injury Studies, which are often cited as rationale for treatment of TON with megadose steroids, do not demonstrate clearly beneficial outcomes and may not apply to TON. These studies investigated the treatment of steroids for acute brain or spinal cord injury, not specifically TON. The most convincing benefit was seen in the group treated with megadoses of steroids (30 mg/kg followed by a continuous infusion of 5.4 mg/kg/h for 24 or 48 hours) within 8 hours of injury, although even this benefit may not be statistically significant. Importantly, there is some evidence that steroids may be detrimental. Optic nerve damage has been shown to worsen with steroid administration in animal models. Additionally, results from the Corticosteroid Randomisation After Significant Head Injury (CRASH) study suggest that high-dose steroids are associated with increased mortality when given in the context of head injury. This large, randomized, placebo-controlled study investigated outcomes following mega-dose steroid treatment (2 g loading dose followed by 0.4 g/hr over 48 hrs) versus placebo in 10,008 patients who had suffered significant head injury. The overall mortality rate 2 weeks following the injury was 21.1% in the steroid group and 17.9% in the placebo group (p=.0001). This refutes previous smaller studies that had suggested decreased mortality following steroid treatment for head injury.

As there is no current standard of care for the treatment of TON, the following options could be offered in the context of the nonrigorous evidence supporting the efficacy of steroid treatment, the greater likelihood of benefit from megadose steroids if given within the 8-hour window following injury, and the possible deleterious effect of this treatment. Moderate dose steroids (250 mg methylprednisolone qid for 24 to 48 hrs) are a reasonable approach, with the theoretic rationale that improvement may result through reduction of edema. Observation or lower dose steroids (100 mg qd) are also reasonable options. Megadose steroids (15 to 30 mg/kg/6 hrs) may be cautiously considered in rare cases, but only if initiated within 8 hours of injury and with the understanding that the risk/benefit ratio is unclear. Optic canal decompression may be indicated when there is radiologic evidence of a bony fragment or hematoma impinging on the optic nerve. It can also be considered in cases of severe vision loss, cases in which surgery is being done to repair other facial fractures, or in cases of continued visual deterioration despite steroid treatment, but only in patients who are conscious and can understand the potential risks and benefits of this procedure that has unproven efficacy. In general, I discourage any treatment beyond moderate doses of steroids in most cases, and particularly in any patient in whom there is diagnostic ambiguity, such as those with simultaneous globe injury or those with severe head injuries that make it difficult to perform a detailed eye examination.

Summary

* TON is a clinical diagnosis.
* CT scan may show a optic canal fracture, orbital fracture, bony fragment, or a sheath or orbital hematoma that might be surgical considerations.
* There are no randomized clinical trial data to provide evidence-based recommendations for treatment of TON.
* Corticosteroids could be considered but are unproven and risk-to-benefit analysis has to be considered.

Bibliography

Bracken MB, Holford TR. Effects of timing of methylprednisolone or naloxone administration on recovery of segmental and long-tract neurological function in NASCIS 2. *Neurosurg.* 1993;79:500-507.

Bracken MB, Shepard MJ, Collins WF, al e. A randomized, controlled trial of methylprednisolone or naloxone in the treatment of acute spinal-cord injury: results of the Second National Acute Spinal Cord Injury Study. *N Engl J Med.* 1990;322(20):1405-1411.

Bracken MB, Shepard MJ, Holford TR, et al. Administration of methylprednisolone for 24 or 48 hours or tirilazad mesylate for 48 hours in the treatment of acute spinal cord injury: results of the Third National Acute Spinal Cord Injury Randomized Controlled Trial. ational Acute Spinal Cord Injury. *JAMA.* 1997;277:1597-1604.

Coleman WP, Benzel D, Cahill DW, et al. A critical appraisal of the reporting of the National Acute Spinal Cord Injury Studies (II and III) of methylprednisolone in acute spinal cord injury. *J Spinal Disord.* 2000;13:185-199.

Diem R, Hobom M, Maier K, et al. Methylprednisolone increases neuronal apoptosis during autoimmune CNS inflammation by inhibition of an endogenous neuroprotective pathway. *J Neurosci.* 2003;23:6993-7000.

Roberts I, Yates D, Sandercock P, et al. Effect of intravenous corticosteroids on death within 14 days in 10008 adults with clinically significant head injury (MRC CRASH trial): randomized placebo-controlled trial. *Lancet.* 2004;364:1321-1328.Steinsapir KD. Treatment of traumatic optic neuropathy with high-dose corticosteroid. *J Neuroophthalmol.* 2006;26(1):65-67.

Steinsapir KD, Goldberg RA. Traumatic optic neuropathy: a critical update. *Compr Ophthalmol Update.* 2005;6(1):11-21.

Steinsapir KD, Goldberg RA, Sinha S, et al. Methylprednisolone exacerbates axonal loss following optic nerve trauma in rats. *Restor Neurol Neurosci.* 2000;17:157-163.

Volpe NJ. Comments on: traumatic optic neuropathy: a critical update. *Compr Ophthalmol Update.* 2005;6(1):23.

11

WHAT IS THE EVALUATION AND MANAGEMENT FOR PAPILLEDEMA?

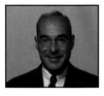

Michael Wall, MD

The patient is a 24-year-old obese female with visual acuity 20/20 OU, perimetry showing only enlarged blind spots, and bilateral papilledema. How do I establish the diagnosis of idiopathic intracranial hypertension (IIH)? What treatments should be started if any? How often should I see this patient? Should I refer this patient to a neurologist?

I would recommend that the modified Dandy criteria should be met for the diagnosis of pseudotumor cerebri or IIH (Table 11-1). The patient should first demonstrate the signs and symptoms of increased intracranial pressure. Headache, transient visual obscurations, pulse synchronous tinnitus, papilledema with associated visual loss, and diplopia due to VI nerve palsies are the common presenting symptoms and signs. An especially important symptom is pulse synchronous tinnitus. This bruit-like sound is present in two-thirds of patients and is rare in the general population, unlike headache. Next, there should be an absence of localized findings on neurologic examination except for the "false localizing" sixth nerve palsies. Neuroimaging should reveal the absence of deformity, displacement, or obstruction of the ventricular system. I like to use magnetic resonance imaging (MRI) and magnetic resonance venography (MRV) in another way. Findings characteristic of increased intracranial pressure are empty sella, smooth walled venous stenoses of the lateral sinuses and orbital findings related to the unfolding of the nerve sheath, and enhancement of the optic disc. Presence of venous sinus collapse (venous stenoses) is especially important, occurring in over 90% of cases when proper MRV is done and can be confused with venous sinus thrombosis. Other neurodiagnostic studies should be normal except for increased cerebrospinal fluid pressure. The patient

---

Table 11-1

Criteria for the Diagnosis of Idiopathic Intracranial Hypertension*

- Signs and symptoms of increased intracranial pressure
- Absence of localizing findings on neurologic examination
- Absence of deformity, displacement, or obstruction of the ventricular system, and otherwise normal neurodiagnostic studies, except for increased cerebrospinal fluid pressure
- Awake and alert patient
- No other cause of increased intracranial pressure present

*Modified Dandy Criteria

---

should be awake and alert and no other cause of increased intracranial pressure should be present.

In the literature, many conditions are purportedly associated with IIH, but case-control studies show that many are simply chance associations due to their frequent occurrence in the population that is susceptible to IIH (young women in the childbearing years). For example, pregnancy, irregular menses, and oral contraceptive use are reported associations that have been shown to be due to chance alone. In case-control studies, no significant association is found between IIH and multivitamin, oral contraceptive, or antibiotic use. A case-control study has found strong associations between IIH, obesity, and weight gain during the 12 months before diagnosis. The interested reader can review a critically evaluated list of conditions and associations of intracranial hypertension.

Your patient sounds like the typical IIH phenotype and is of the characteristic age. We should proceed to see if she fulfills the modified Dandy criteria for IIH. If she has typical symptoms of increased intracranial pressure, clear findings of obvious papilledema, MRI with characteristic abnormalities, normal cerebrospinal fluid (CSF) pressure except for a high opening pressure, and no other cause of intracranial hypertension apparent, I would not go further since there is little uncertainty. However, with the presence of diagnostic uncertainty (eg, if the patient is a male), more testing (eg, MRV or an evaluation for sleep apnea) is performed.

Let us presume this is a typical presentation for IIH so we then start treatment. I typically treat all patients with a low-sodium weight management program. Patients usually improve with weight loss of 5% to 10% body weight. Much more weight loss usually is not sustainable and does not appear to be necessary for IIH remission. Weight loss may be all our patient needs since there is no visual loss with perimetric examination except for enlarged blind spots. However, if her symptoms of intracranial hypertension were interfering with her activities of daily living (eg, severe headache), I would start acetazolamide in gradually escalating doses to 1 to 2 g per day. Lasix can be used if the patient cannot tolerate acetazolamide. Topiramate does not appear to be any more efficacious than acetazolamide. However, all reports of treatment of IIH are anecdotal and uncontrolled.

The frequency of follow-up depends mostly on risk of visual loss. The 2 most important factors here are amount of visual loss present and the degree of optic disc edema. If

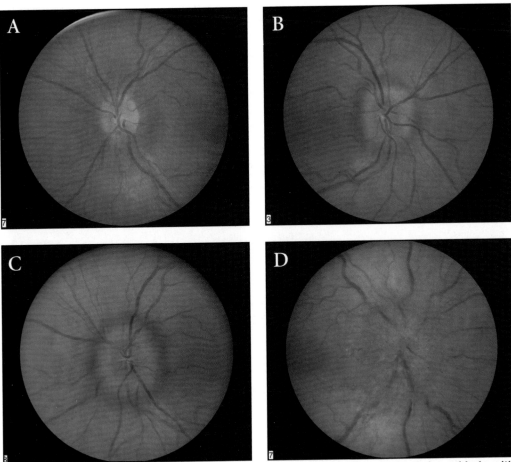

Figure 11-1. An example of Frisén grades for optic disc edema. (A) Note the C-shaped halo with a temporal gap in Grade 1. (B) There is Grade 2 (360 degrees) of disc edema. (C) In Grade 3 disc edema there is obscuration of the peripapillary major blood vessel as it crosses the disc margin. (D) In Grade 4 optic disc edema there is obscuration of the major blood vessel in the center of the disc.

the risk of further visual loss is low, the usual revisit time after diagnosis is 1 to 2 months. I would have this patient back in 2 months and, if she is doing well, again in 4 months. Since IIH can be a lifelong disease (like arterial hypertension), I follow patients who are in remission every 1 to 2 years. The key features when following a patient are the change in weight, change in symptoms, perimetry results, and papilledema grade (Figure 11-1). I also grade optic discs using the Frisén scale—a monocular-based, graded staging scheme that is descriptive in nature—and take optic disc photos when changes occur. Diagnosis and treatment should be done either by an ophthalmologist and neurologist working together or ideally by a neuro-ophthalmologist. Complicated cases should be managed by a neuro-ophthalmologist.

Summary

* IIH is a diagnosis of exclusion (modified Dandy criteria).

* The typical patient with IIH is an overweight young female, and more aggressive evaluation for possible etiologies should be considered in thin patients, men, and the elderly.

* Medical treatment with weight loss and acetazolamide are the first lines of therapy.

* Surgical treatment (optic nerve sheath fenestration or shunting procedures) are reserved for patients with progressive disease who fail maximum medical therapy.

Bibliography

Farb RI, Vanek I, Scott JN, et al. Idiopathic intracranial hypertension: the prevalence and morphology of sinovenous stenosis. *Neurology.* 2003;60:1418-1424.

Giuseffi V, Wall M, Siegel PZ, Rojas PB. Symptoms and disease associations in idiopathic intracranial hypertension (pseudotumor cerebri): a case-control study. *Neurology.* 1991;41:239-244.

Wall M. Papilledema and idiopathic intracranial hypertension (pseudotumor cerebri). In: Noseworthy JH, ed. *Neurological Therapeutics: Principles and Practice.* Abingdon, UK: Informa Healthcare; 2006:1955-1968.

Wall M, George D. Idiopathic intracranial hypertension: a prospective study of 50 patients. *Brain.* 1991;114:155-180.

12

IS THERE A DIFFERENCE IN THE MANAGEMENT OF PSEUDOTUMOR CEREBRI IN PREGNANCY?

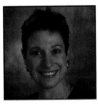

Deborah I. Friedman, MD, FAAN

The patient is a 24-year-old female who is pregnant and has papilledema OU. She has headache but her visual acuity is 20/20 OU and only a big blind spot on her automated visual field testing. Do you do anything differently with your pseudotumor cerebri (PTC) patients who are pregnant? Do you think that this constitutes a "high-risk" pregnancy? Can you use acetazolamide in pregnancy? Can you do serial lumbar punctures in pregnancy? Can she have magnetic resonance imaging (MRI)? Can she have gadolinium contrast with the MRI?

PTC, particular the idiopathic form (ie, idiopathic intracranial hypertension or IIH), most frequently affects young women of childbearing age, so the issue of potential pregnancy often arises. I get emails from women with IIH worldwide asking the same questions. Worse yet, women with IIH are sometimes advised by their physicians to avoid becoming pregnant or to consider having an abortion!

If your patient had IIH prior to becoming pregnant, she will likely do very well during her pregnancy. I generally monitor these patients throughout their pregnancy with examinations and perimetry. Flare-ups can generally be managed with intermittent therapeutic lumbar punctures (pregnancy is one circumstance where serial lumbar punctures are the preferred treatment). Acetazolamide (a US Food and Drug Administration [FDA] category C agent) may be used during pregnancy, although I recommend avoiding it during the first trimester; often the lumbar puncture will buy enough time to accomplish this.

Women may develop IIH for the first time during pregnancy or may have an exacerbation or recurrence of IIH during pregnancy. Diagnosis of IIH during pregnancy is the same as in the nongravid state: neuroimaging (MRI, MR venogram) and lumbar puncture. Gadolinium is a category C agent, however, and some radiologists are hesitant to prescribe it. Make sure that your patient is not taking supplemental vitamin A with her prenatal vitamins. The treatment (ie, avoiding acetazolamide and other diuretics during the first trimester if possible) is also the same. If vision is threatened, optic nerve sheath fenestration or shunting may be performed, keeping in mind that the expanding uterus might potentially impinge on the abdominal end of the shunt catheter.

IIH developing during pregnancy or shortly after delivery should prompt investigations for cerebral venous sinus thrombosis and thrombophilia.

Let us also consider the situation where vision is normal and the main problem is headache. Headaches during pregnancy can be difficult to treat because so many of the preventive and symptomatic headache medications are FDA category C. Vitamin B_2 (riboflavin, 300 mg daily) and magnesium (300 mg daily) may be employed for headache prevention. A low-dose tricyclic antidepressant, such as amitriptyline or nortriptyline, or a selective serotonin reuptake inhibitor (SSRI) may be considered after the first trimester has passed. Valproate and gabapentin are contraindicated, as are the triptans and dihydroergotamine. Acetaminophen with codeine or narcotic analgesics may be sparingly used for symptomatic headache treatment. It is always best to work closely with the patient's obstetrician during the pregnancy, particularly if questions arise about medications that may be used.

IIH does not, in and of itself, define a high-risk pregnancy. Women with IIH may deliver vaginally if there is no obstetrical contraindication, and no special anesthetics are required. A possible exception is the presence of very high-grade papilledema at the time of delivery; pushing during labor could potentially worsen it so a cesarean section might be considered in that circumstance. Fortunately, it is a rare occurrence.

The bottom line is that most women with IIH get through their pregnancies without serious problems. Neither the disease nor the treatment has a harmful effect on the baby. Who knows... she might even name her baby after you!

Summary

* The evaluation and management of IIH in pregnancy and outside of pregnancy are similar (although the suspicion for possible cerebral venous sinus thrombosis should be higher in pregnant or postpartum patients).

* The contrast material in MRI, however, is FDA category C and some radiologists are hesitant to give gadolinium in pregnancy.

* IIH in pregnancy by itself does not define a high-risk pregnancy.

* Acetazolamide is also an FDA category C agent but may be used in pregnancy (although it might be wise to avoid it in the first trimester).

Bibliography

Digre KB, Varner MV, Corbett JJ. Pseudotumor cerebri and pregnancy. *Neurology.* 1984;34:721-729.
Evans RW, Friedman DI. The management of pseudotumor cerebri during pregnancy. *Headache.* 2000;40:496-497.
Huna-Baron R, Kupersmith MJ. Idiopathic intracranial hypertension in pregnancy. *J Neurol.* 2002;249:1078-1081.

13

WHAT IS THE EVALUATION AND MANAGEMENT OF THE HIGH-FLOW CAROTID CAVERNOUS FISTULA?

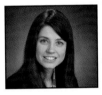

Victoria S. Pelak, MD (co-authored with Drew Dixon, MD)

The patient is a 21-year-old man who sustained closed head trauma in a motor vehicle accident. Over the ensuing week he developed increasing right proptosis with chemosis, lid edema, right limited eye movements in all directions, and a "roaring" sound in his head. What is the most likely diagnosis and how should the patient be evaluated and treated?

There are several features of this clinical presentation that should alert you to a possible direct carotid cavernous fistula (CCF). First, your patient is presenting with orbital signs, which in conjunction with chemosis and periorbital soft tissue edema are suggestive of orbital congestion. Your patient is also complaining of a "roaring" sound in his head, which is concerning for a high-flow vascular abnormality. Lastly, there is a history of recent head injury, and that is a common risk factor for direct carotid cavernous sinus fistula formation.

Carotid cavernous sinus fistulae are generally classified into 2 broad groups based on angiographic findings: 1) direct and 2) indirect. All CCF represent an abnormal anastomosis between the high-flow arterial system of the carotid arteries and the relatively low-flow venous system of the cavernous sinus. A direct CCF, as its name suggests, is a direct connection between the intracavernous internal carotid artery and the cavernous sinus. The most common cause of direct CCF is a traumatic tear in the wall of the intracavernous carotid artery in the setting of head trauma (approximately 75% of all CCF), typically in young males (Figures 13-1 and 13-2). Rarely, direct CCF can occur from spontaneous aneurysm rupture in the presence of underlying collagen vascular disease. Indirect CCFs are generally low-flow shunts formed between the cavernous sinus and

Figure 13-1. A 19-year-old man who presented 3 days following a motor vehicle accident with near complete ophthalmoplegia and ptosis of the right due to a high-flow CCF. In all positions of gaze, forced duction testing (only left gaze is shown) revealed restriction, implicating involvement of the third, fourth, and sixth nerves in addition to

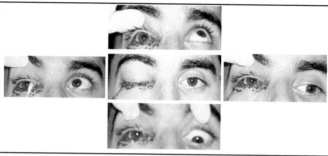

congested extraocular muscles (also seen on MR orbit but not shown here) as cause for the ophthalmoplegia.

Figure 13-2. (A) Lateral view of right carotid angiogram of patient shown in Figure 13-1. The high-flow CCF can be seen with flow from the cavernous carotid directly into the superior ophthalmic vein (open block arrow) and inferior ophthalmic vein (closed block arrow). Flow during the arterial phase continues from the orbital veins to facial vein (small arrow) and

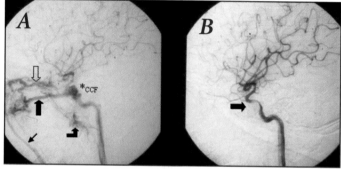

pterygoid plexus (bent arrow). (B) Same patient following embolization of the CCF with coiling (black arrow). No flow into the ophthalmic or facial veins or pterygoid plexus during arterial phase is seen and the carotid artery remains patent with improved flow into cerebral branches.

dural branches of either the internal or external carotid arteries. We find the symptoms at presentation can vary considerably and depend upon the size of the fistula, duration of the lesion, and direction of venous drainage. Fistulas may drain either anteriorly into the ophthalmic veins or posteriorly into the petrosal sinuses. It is important to be aware that fistulae that drain posteriorly may not present with classic findings. Morbidity from CCF is caused by both venous congestion and a lack of blood flow to ocular structures as a result of shunting.

Direct CCF typically presents more acutely, usually within days to weeks of an inciting trauma, as opposed to weeks to months for indirect CCF. Rapidly progressive proptosis over the course of hours is unusual and may represent thrombosis of the orbital venous outflow system, which requires urgent evaluation and intervention. Direct CCFs are also more likely to present with the classic triad of chemosis, pulsatile exophthalmos, and ocular bruit compared to indirect CCF. In addition to the classic triad, external examination may show eyelid edema, dilated conjunctival vessels, exposure keratopathy, and limited extraocular movements (see Figure 13-1). Dilated funduscopic examination can demonstrate intraretinal hemorrhages, vitreous hemorrhage, dilated retinal veins, optic disc swelling, proliferative retinopathy, or central retinal vein occlusion. Intraocular pressure can be elevated, as both neovascular glaucoma and angle-closure glaucoma (secondary to choroidal congestion and anterior displacement of the lens-iris diaphragm) have been reported. Vision loss at presentation occurs in approximately 20% to 35% of patients and may result from any of the above processes, including ischemia of the optic nerve. One of the most devastating complications of direct CCF is hemorrhage. Both intracranial hemorrhage and severe epistaxis have been reported in the literature, including cases resulting in death. For this reason we always ask patients about neurologic symptoms related to these lesions and perform a full neurological examination immediately.

In our opinion, both computed tomography (CT) and magnetic resonance imaging (MRI) scans of the orbits are useful initial screening examinations. Both studies can demonstrate findings suggestive of a CCF or alternative causes for the patient's presentation, although MRI is more useful in identifying the degree of associated cerebral parenchymal injury. Radiographic findings in the setting of CCF may include orbital edema, enlargement of the ipsilateral cavernous sinus, proptosis, and enlargement of the ipsilateral superior ophthalmic vein. As a general rule of thumb, an asymmetric superior ophthalmic vein or a vein larger than 4 mm probably represents pathologic enlargement; MRI of the orbit is best to accurately measure vein size. It is important to note that an asymmetric superior ophthalmic vein is not a specific finding and can be seen in other orbital pathologies such as orbit vascular malformations. However, with an appropriate history, an enlarged superior ophthalmic vein is highly suggestive of an indirect or direct CCF. As mentioned previously, some fistulae drain primarily posteriorly into the petrosal sinuses, and in these instances, the superior ophthalmic vein may not be enlarged. If the diagnosis is still uncertain or the patient's symptoms do not warrant intervention, we typically perform a CT angiogram (CTA) to help confirm the diagnosis and define the anatomy. CTA is less invasive than digital subtraction cerebral angiography, yet still provides detail about the size and location of the fistula. Other noninvasive techniques for assessing CCF include MR angiogram (MRA) and Doppler ultrasound. CTA is generally better at characterizing fistula anatomy than MRA, especially segment 4 of the internal carotid artery, which is the location of approximately half of all direct CCF. Doppler ultrasound, while able to accurately diagnose both high- and low-flow lesions, requires a skilled technician and does not provide precise details of size and location.

If the patient's symptoms warrant intervention, catheter angiography should be performed. Digital subtraction cerebral angiography is the most common modality used and is necessary to define anatomy before and during embolization (see Figure 13-2). The goal of treatment is to close the fistula while maintaining patency of the internal carotid artery. Most commonly, embolization is achieved utilizing detachable balloons or coils. The reported success rate for embolization ranges from 89% to 99%.

If you suspect your patient has a direct or indirect CCF, further imaging will lead to proper assessment and treatment of the condition. Early recognition is a key to preventing ophthalmic and neurologic morbidity and, in rare instances, mortality.

Bibliography

Chen CC, Chang PC, Shy CG, Chen WS, Hung HC. CT angiography and MR angiography in the evaluation of carotid cavernous sinus fistula prior to embolization: a comparison of techniques. *Am J Neuroradiol.* 2005;26:2349-2356.

Fleishman JA, Garfinkel RA, Beck RW. Advances in the treatment of carotid cavernous fistula. *Int Ophthalmol Clin.* 1986;26:301-311.

Gupta AK, Purkayastha S, Krishnamoorthy T, et al. Endovascular treatment of direct carotid cavernous fistulae: a pictorial review. *Neuroradiology.* 2006;48:831-839.

Harris GJ, Rice PR. Angle closure in carotid-cavernous fistula. *Ophthalmology*. 1979;86:1521-1529.
Sugar HS. Neovascular glaucoma after carotid-cavernous fistula formation. *Ann Ophthalmol*. 1979;11:1667-1669.

How Do I Manage an
Internuclear Ophthalmoplegia?

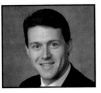

Christopher C. Glisson, DO
(co-authored with David I. Kaufman, DO)

A 45-year-old patient has double vision. Examination reveals impairment of adduction in the left eye with nystagmus in the right eye on right lateral gaze. How is internuclear ophthalmoplegia (INO) proven? Can it be anything else? What is the work-up for an INO?

The examination findings describe a common presentation of INO—impaired adduction of one eye associated with monocular nystagmus in the contralateral (abducting) eye. However, confidence in the diagnosis rests upon a careful consideration of the patient's history, followed by a detailed examination to document the presence (or absence) of any associated features. By this approach, the site of the lesion can be exquisitely localized, alternate etiologies (or "mimics") can be considered, and the appropriate diagnostic testing can be obtained.

Patients with an isolated INO may be asymptomatic. Alternatively, asymmetry in the speed of horizontal saccades between the abducting and adducting eye can give the brief sensation of disparate images that "have to catch up to each other." Other patients may report horizontal double vision. Overall, INO can precipitate a continuum of visual disturbances—ranging from blurring to overt diplopia—as a consequence of adduction weakness or skew deviation. Oscillopsia of one image (due to abduction nystagmus) may also be described.

On examination, the presence of an INO is suggested by unilateral adduction weakness in conjunction with abduction nystagmus in the fellow eye. These findings are best elicited by testing saccades rather than smooth pursuit movements, as the medial longitudinal fasciculus (MLF) mainly carries fibers relaying the "pulse" of the saccade rather

---

Table 14-1

Most Common Causes of Internuclear Ophthalmoplegia

Above Age 45
- Ischemia
- Multiple sclerosis
- Tumor (primary or metastatic)

Below Age 45
- Multiple sclerosis
- Trauma
- Tumor (primary or metastatic)
- Ischemia

Adapted from Lavin PJM, Donahue SP. Neuro-ophthalmology: ocular motor system. In: Bradley WG, Daroff RJ, Fenichel GM, Jankovic J, eds. *Neurology in Clinical Practice: Principles of Diagnosis and Management.* 4th ed. Philadelphia, PA: Elsevier; 2004:718 and Keane JR. Internuclear ophthalmoplegia: unusual cases in 114 of 410 patients. *Arch Neurol.* 2005;62:714-717.

---

than the "step" of smooth pursuit. Large-amplitude saccades and random targets also increase the yield of testing for an INO.

The hallmark of INO is "adduction lag" of the eye ipsilateral to the site of the lesion. Appreciation of a subtle adduction lag may be enhanced through the use of an optokinetic drum, which allows the amplitude and velocity of saccades in each eye to be compared, thus emphasizing the slowed adduction of the affected eye. Other examination features may include skew deviation (usually with hypertropia ipsilateral to the adduction lag), impaired vertical vestibulo-ocular reflex, and impaired vertical smooth pursuit.

INO results from a lesion involving the MLF, a paired fiber tract that transmits neural impulses from the sixth nerve nucleus to the contralateral third nerve nucleus. Disruption of the MLF (by any mechanism, see below) impairs the pathway mediating conjugate eye movements within the horizontal plane by effectively limiting input to the medial rectus muscle ipsilateral to the lesion. The contralateral eye develops nystagmus in abduction. This nystagmus is likely a reflection of Hering's law, with equal innervation to the yoked horizontal eye muscles in the face of impaired adduction but full abduction.

Numerous causes of INO have been reported in the literature. However, in practice, the most common causes are really quite few in number (Table 14-1). If the INO is an isolated finding, the primary differential diagnosis can be based on the patient's age. From 18 to 45 years, demyelination is most frequent; in patients older than 45, stroke (including vertebral artery dissection) followed by demyelination should be regarded as the most likely cause.

INO may be unilateral or bilateral, reflecting involvement of one or both MLFs. A bilateral INO is most classically associated with multiple sclerosis (MS) in the appropriate age group. However, systemic processes such as metabolic and nutritional derangements can result in bilateral involvement. Wall-eyed binocular INO (WEBINO) syndrome results from bilateral MLF lesions, with resultant exotropia in primary position. The unilateral or bilateral nature of INO is not consistent among etiologies, and so should not be used as a definitive diagnostic feature. There are variations of INO that can also help with localization, including the one-and-a-half syndrome (a lesion of the caudal dorsal pontine tegmentum and ipsilateral MLF, with only abduction of one eye remaining intact), and the eight-and-a-half syndrome (one-and-a-half plus cranial nerve VII palsy, often due to pontine ischemia).

Patients with INO should be evaluated based on their clinical history and examination, and investigations should be guided by accurate localization of the presumptive lesion causing the adduction deficit. In most instances, thin slice (2 to 3 mm) magnetic resonance imaging (MRI) of the brain with gadolinium is required. Confirmatory findings at imaging should include involvement of the dorsal aspect of the caudal pons, ipsilateral to the impaired adduction. It should be noted that an abnormality is not always documented even on thin slice MRI. MRI also allows the opportunity to investigate for MS, acute stroke, and other unexpected causes (such as an orbital or third nerve mass or thyroid eye disease).

In the appropriate clinical setting, additional diagnostic studies directed toward alternative causes of INO (see Table 14-1) should be undertaken. If pseudo-INO from ocular myasthenia is suspected, a "rest test" can be performed. If there is improvement in ocular motility after 10 to 15 minutes of rest, the observed motility deficit is possibly due to myasthenia gravis. Prostigmin and Tensilon (Valeant Pharmaceuticals International, Aliso Viejo, CA) could also be considered. Thyroid eye disease may be associated with proptosis or lid lag. A partial third nerve palsy due to a compressive lesion may be associated with aberrant regeneration involving the pupil or eyelid.

Finally, the presence of an INO in people under the age of 45 necessitates a discussion related to possible MS and the need to pursue that diagnosis with MRI and other studies to see if immunomodulating agents seem logical. Over the age of 45, risk factors for stroke and also MS should be reviewed and evaluated, with appropriate therapy considered in confirmed cases of these diseases.

Summary

* Internuclear ophthalmoplegia (INO) results from a lesion of the ipsilateral medial longitudinal fasciculus (MLF).
* Patients with INO may be asymptomatic, or may describe blurred vision or diplopia.
* INO is recognized clinically by adduction lag in one eye, classically associated with abduction nystagmus in the fellow eye.
* In patients aged 18-45, demyelination is the most common cause of INO.
* In patients older than age 45, stroke and MS are the most common causes of INO.
* Magnetic resonance imaging (MRI) is recommended to evaluate for the causes (and mimics) of INO, including multiple sclerosis, stroke, mass and thyroid eye disease.

Bibliography

Eggenberger E. Eight-and-a-half-syndrome: one-and-a-half plus cranial nerve VII palsy. *J Neuroophthalmol.* 1998; 18(2):114-116.

Keane JR. Internuclear ophthalmoplegia: unusual cases in 114 of 410 patients. *Arch Neurol.* 2005;62:714-717.

Leigh RJ, Zee DS. *The Neurology of Eye Movements.* 4th ed. New York: Oxford University Press, 2006.

Wall M, Wray SH. The one-and-a-half syndrome: a unilateral disorder of the pontine tegmentum. *Neurology.* 1983; 33:971.

WHAT IS THE EVALUATION OF OCULAR MYASTHENIA GRAVIS?

Laura J. Balcer MD, MSCE
(co-authored with Raymond Price, MD)

The patient is a 29-year-old woman with isolated ocular myasthenia gravis and I was wondering what you thought the best evaluation and treatment options are for ocular myasthenia gravis. Could you tell me how to confirm the diagnosis and how, when, and why should treatment be given for ocular myasthenia gravis?

There are 2 major types of myasthenia gravis: generalized and isolated ocular (15% of cases). In isolated ocular myasthenia gravis, patients describe some combination of fluctuating ptosis and diplopia that increases as the day progresses and with sustained activity. They should not report or subsequently develop dysarthria, dysphagia, head drop, shortness of breath, or difficulty rising from a chair. On physical examination, patients will have fluctuating unilateral or bilateral ptosis, worsened by prolonged upgaze or by elevation of the contralateral eyelid (curtaining), and fluctuating ocular misalignment in the horizontal or vertical plane. They should not have or develop facial weakness, dysarthria, or weakness on confrontational testing of neck, shoulder, and hip flexion.

The distinction between generalized and isolated ocular myasthenia is quite clear with a few years of serial evaluations but may be impossible to make at initial presentation. More than half of the patients with myasthenia gravis will present with ocular signs and symptoms only. Most patients (94%) with generalized myasthenia gravis, who presented with ocular signs and symptoms, will develop nonocular weakness within 3 years of presentation.

At the initial office visit, you may be tempted to confirm the diagnosis of myasthenia gravis with either the icepack or Tensilon test. Although some authors believe strongly in these diagnostic clinical tests, our experience has been that they are less useful. The icepack test can only be used to evaluate a prominent ptosis and cannot be used for ocular misalignment. Similar improvement in ptosis may occur with heat and sleep, and thus some authors argue that the icepack test is only evaluating rest. Both tests are relatively sensitive; 80% for an icepack test and 85% to 95% for the Tensilon test with a measurable ptosis or ocular misalignment, but their specificity and predictive value are unclear. We would recommend deferring these tests unless the results of either test would alter your working diagnosis or evaluation. In cases where the diagnosis is clear or the patient has other risk factors, we normally skip the pharmacologic testing as the Tensilon test is not without risk. There is the small potential risk for cardiac arrhythmias, including asystole. Some authors have used Prostigmin (Valeant Pharmaceuticals, Aliso Viejo, CA) (as it is longer lasting) for ophthalmoplegia, but we have less experience or recommendations for this pharmacologic test.

Instead, we would recommend performing a thorough evaluation to both exclude alternative etiologies and confirm the diagnosis of myasthenia gravis. Although many diseases can present with weakness of the muscles typically affected in myasthenia gravis, the fluctuating nature of this weakness is relatively specific for a disorder of neuromuscular transmission. If the patient presents with isolated ocular symptoms, one could consider a sellar lesion such as a meningioma or aneurysm, and a brainstem lesion, which can be excluded by magnetic resonance imaging (MRI) of the brain with thin slices through the sella and magnetic resonance angiography (MRA) of the head. In cases of clear cut myasthenia gravis however imaging is generally not necessary. Strictly unilateral patients, however, might require imaging especially if the other testing is negative (eg, antibody testing, pharmacologic testing).

Other etiologies for diplopia or ophthalmoplegia include chronic progressive external ophthalmoplegia and oculopharyngeal muscular dystrophy, which can be evaluated by electrophysiologic testing (eg, electromyogram [EMG]). If the patient presents with more generalized weakness, one should also consider the less common etiologies (eg, botulism, Lambert-Eaton myasthenic syndrome, polymyositis, myotonic dystrophy, and mitochondrial myopathy), all of which can also be evaluated by an EMG.

There are a number of available tests to confirm a diagnosis of isolated ocular myasthenia gravis. Serum testing for antibodies against the neuromuscular junction and special EMG testing remain the standard for confirmation of myasthenia gravis. Both of these tests are more useful for generalized myasthenia gravis than isolated ocular myasthenia gravis. The first confirmatory test that I send is the acetylcholine receptor antibody. Some authors only perform the screening antibody testing (eg, binding), but others recommend testing for all 3 antibodies (eg, binding, blocking, and modulating). The sensitivity and specificity for antibodies against the acetylcholine receptor in isolated ocular myasthenia gravis are 45% to 60% and 100%, respectively. There are only a few case reports of antibodies against the muscle specific tyrosine-kinase (MuSK) in isolated ocular myasthenia gravis and therefore it should not be routinely ordered.

If the acetylcholine receptor antibody is negative but the suspicion for myasthenia gravis remains high, I would consider a repetitive nerve stimulation and single-fiber EMG. Repetitive nerve stimulation of multiple sites is only 33% to 45% sensitive and 89% specific in isolated ocular myasthenia. Single-fiber EMG is the best available test for myasthenia gravis. If the superior rectus and levator palpebrae are evaluated, the sensitivity of single-fiber EMG for isolated ocular myasthenia has been reported at greater than 95%.

While many muscle diseases can produce an abnormal single-fiber EMG, the specificity of single-fiber EMG is quite high in the appropriate clinical context of fluctuating weakness. The limiting factor for single-fiber EMG is its availability.

Once the diagnosis of myasthenia gravis is established, computed tomography (CT) of the chest should be performed to exclude a thymoma. Thirty percent to 40% of thymomas are locally invasive and termed *malignant,* but metastases are rare. If a thymoma is present, the patient should be referred for thymectomy. Thymectomy for the treatment of isolated ocular myasthenia in the absence of a thymoma remains controversial. A recent case series suggested a symptomatic benefit following thymectomy in ocular myasthenia, but these benefits need to be balanced against the risk of surgery.

Symptomatic relief can be provided without medications by lid adhesives for ptosis or an eye patch or opaque lens for diplopia. In our experience, eyelid crutches do not usually provide adequate symptomatic relief. If patients choose either eyelid crutches or lid adhesives for ptosis, they must be informed of the risk of corneal damage from constant exposure and be treated with frequent ocular lubrication.

If a patient is not satisfied with nonpharmacological treatments, a trial of pyridostigmine should be offered. To minimize the cholinergic side effects of pyridostigmine, especially diarrhea, patients should take an antimuscarinic medication such as glycopyrrolate. Unfortunately, the likelihood of symptomatic relief with pyridostigmine alone is low, only 6.9% in one case series.

In contrast, corticosteroids can be a highly effective treatment for isolated ocular myasthenia gravis. In one case series, 70% of patients treated with prednisone achieved symptomatic relief in one month that was maintained at 2 years. If symptomatic relief can not be achieved with pyridostigmine, the risks and benefits of chronic corticosteroid treatment should be discussed with the patient. Other immunosuppressive medications such as azathioprine, mycophenolate, and cyclosporine may be beneficial for symptomatic relief but their use is limited by their side effect profile. Use of these medications must be made on a case to case basis. Currently, there is no randomized controlled evidence that chronic immunosuppression has any benefit at preventing isolated ocular myasthenia from progressing to generalized myasthenia. A trial addressing this question is currently underway. If a patient develops generalized myasthenia, he or she should be treated with chronic immunosuppression and pyridostigmine for symptomatic relief. Ten percent of patients with isolated ocular myasthenia gravis will have spontaneously remission of their symptoms without treatment.

Summary

* In the setting of isolated ocular myasthenia:
  * The initial evaluation includes clinical evaluation, consideration for pharmacologic or other adjunctive testing, and anti-acetylcholine receptor antibody tests. If the acetylcholine antibody testing is negative, a single-fiber EMG could be performed but may not be universally available. A CT scan of the chest should be performed to exclude an underlying thymoma. Neuroimaging studies are generally not needed for typical myasthenia gravis confirmed clinically, pharmacologically, or serologically but should be considered in atypical cases (eg, strictly unilateral findings without other confirmatory evidence for myasthenia gravis).

❖ Symptomatic relief should be offered to all patients. Therapeutic options include both nonpharmacologic interventions such as eyelid crutches or an eye patch and pharmacologic treatment with pyridostigmine and glycopyrrolate.

❖ Corticosteroids are likely to provide symptomatic relief but with the associated side effects of chronic steroid use. The use of corticosteroids must be individualized to the patient who has persistent symptoms despite pyridostigmine.

❖ Alternative immunosuppressive medications and thymectomy may be considered in some cases and must be individualized to the patient after a thorough discussion of the potential risks of treatment.

❖ Currently, there is no proven benefit of chronic immunosuppression for the prevention of disease progression.

❖ Exacerbating medications should be avoided.

Bibliography

Costa J, Evangelista T, Conceicao I, de Carvalho M. Repetitive nerve stimulation in myasthenia gravis--relative sensitivity of different muscles. *Clin Neurophysiol.* 2004;115:2776-2782.

Elrod RD, Weinberg DA. Ocular myasthenia gravis. *Ophthalmol Clin North Am.* 2004;17:275-309; v.

Golnik KC, Pena R, Lee AG, Eggenberger ER. An ice test for the diagnosis of myasthenia gravis. *Ophthalmology.* 1999;106:1282-1286.

Meriggioli MN, Sanders DB. Myasthenia gravis: diagnosis. *Semin Neurol.* 2004;24:31-39.

Valls-Canals J, Povedano M, Montero J, Pradas J. Stimulated single-fiber EMG of the frontalis and orbicularis oculi muscles in ocular myasthenia gravis. *Muscle Nerve.* 2003;28:501-503.

WHAT DO I TELL MY PATIENTS WITH OCULAR MYASTHENIA ABOUT THEIR CHANCES OF IT PROGRESSING TO THE REST OF THEIR BODY? DO I NEED A NEUROLOGIST?

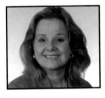

Pamela S. Chavis, MD
(co-authored with Peter Savino, MD)

The patient is a 45-year-old man with proven ocular myasthenia gravis (OMG). What are his chances of developing generalized myasthenia gravis (GMG)? How likely do you think it is for a patient with OMG to develop generalized symptoms and what problems could occur? Are there other medicines he should avoid?

The majority of patients with myasthenia will present with the ocular findings and the odds are that 20% to 40% of patients will remain ocular. If their disease persists as ocular for 2 years, then 90% will not further generalize. The remaining 60% to 80% of patients who do not remain ocular might require therapeutic medical and/or surgical intervention but today can generally expect an excellent outcome. However, there are 4 outcome modifiers for the GMG group: 1) rapid progression of systemic weakness, 2) severely impaired respiratory function, 3) thymoma, and 4) autoimmune disease. For these reasons we do believe that ophthalmologists should consult a colleague in neurology or neuro-ophthalmology for their OMG patients.

The consulting neurologist or neuro-ophthalmologist might consider a number of additional tests for the evaluation of pernicious anemia: antinuclear antibody (ANA), rheumatoid factor, myasthenia antibody panel, anti-MuSK antibodies, Tensilon or Prostigmin test; renal function:computed contrast tomography of the chest (eg, thymoma or thymic hyperplasia); thyroid function tests; pulmonary function tests; or repetitive electromyography stimulation (particularly single fiber).

About 10% of ocular myasthenia patients will experience a spontaneous remission. The patient with pure ocular involvement has options unless there is thymoma or autoimmune disease involvement, since these will require direct intervention. To some degree, the intervention is balanced by the degree of ocular involvement, age, comorbidity, and lifestyle. A patient with minimal involvement can be observed, while disease progression with accompanying lifestyle impact is assessed, because symptomatic ocular progression usually happens within the first 3 to 4 years of the disease.

Anticholinesterase agents are most effective for fatiguing ptosis. While the usual starting dose of pyridostigmine is 60 mg 3 times daily, each dose is metabolized completely in 4 hours. Hence, a starting dose that ensures a more even titration may be achieved by 30 mg every 3 hours (5 to 6 doses) while awake (a pre-nap or bedtime dose is not necessary). Subsequent titration depends upon patient response, which can be assessed by a patient diary and outpatient visits in the afternoon. Systemic effects are usually gastric distress and diarrhea, which can be handled with reassurance and specific therapy; muscle cramps may occur but are neither severe nor ominous. Oral atropine can ameliorate some side effects but it is usually not necessary at standard doses for OMG. Since the extraocular muscle(s) involvement can be variable and asymmetric, it is more difficult to treat diplopia effectively with pyridostigmine. Assistive devices such as Fresnel prisms will be helpful if the extraocular muscle involvement is minimal and stable; lid crutches for ptosis usually are not tolerated.

It has been my practice to perform skin testing for latent tuberculosis at the initiation of steroid treatment, but this is not a universal recommendation. In addition, high-dose steroids can produce a paradoxical severe weakness and respiratory collapse so it has been preferred to introduce steroids slowly at the rate of 10 to 20 mg daily (or on alternate days in mild cases). This is increased by 5 to 10 mg daily every 5 to 7 days until clinical improvement or a dose of 60 mg occurs. It is certainly important to alert the patient of concerns for additional or sudden weakness, but most tolerate this slower induction well. Hand-held plastic tidal volume measures (such as are used at home by asthmatics) are optional but not essential. When the patient is stable for at least 3 months, the dose can be gradually reduced in 5-mg increments to a low maintenance dose of 7.5 to 12.5 mg daily or alternate day dosing of 10 to 15 mg. Clinical responses usually are apparent within 2 to 4 weeks with maximum benefit occurring by 6 to 12 months. If symptoms recur, then the dose can be increased by 10- to 20-mg increments each week until the patient is clinically improved again.

Corticosteroid use becomes an important consideration due to potential life-threatening problems such as respiratory impairment, which occurs with GMG. Dysphagia bulbi especially for liquids is an alerting sign of bulbar and potential respiratory involvement; solids and semi-solids may descend more easily through the esophagus with less muscle coordination required. Early treatment with corticosteroids might reduce the rate of progression to GMG although this still remains a bit controversial. Studies where treatment was started more than 1 year after disease presentation have shown less clear results. Subsequent exacerbations may occur despite any therapy and require retreatment in many patients until their therapy has been individualized successfully.

The risks of steroids include Cushing-like changes, diabetes mellitus, hypertension, gastric ulceration, proximal muscle weakness, infections, cataracts, and osteoporosis. The patient and his or her primary care physician can help monitor blood pressure, diet control, and physical therapy for proximal muscles. Osteoporosis and gastric mucosal changes can be anticipated and patients treated during steroid therapy. Dosing must be slowly tapered to alternate days to minimize the risk of adrenal insufficiency. However, in OMG patients in whom steroids were ineffective or cannot be used, other agents such as azathioprine and mycophenolate mofetil have been well-tolerated and effective; thymectomy has also had favorable results in some OMG studies. Cyclosporine as an immunostatic anti-T-cell agent has such renal and hepatic effects that it is only used as later and alternative treatment. Intravenous immunoglobulin has been helpful in juvenile MG or in GMG where steroids have not been tolerated.

The list of drugs or agents that could be *avoided if possible* in myasthenia patients is long. It includes the statins and possibly gabapentin, which may uncover latent myasthenia, as well as D-penicillamine, which induces MG. It also includes all the "–mycin" antibiotics, aminoglycosides, tetracycline, ciprofloxacin, bacitracin, beta-blockers (including topical), calcium channel-blockers, quinine, anti-arrhythmias, lithium, chloroquine, respiratory depressants, magnesium sulfate, and neuromuscular blockers.

Summary

* OMG should probably be managed by an ophthalmologist in conjunction with a neurologist or neuro-ophthalmologist.

* Generalization of OMG to systemic MG is common but typically occurs in the first 2 years following the diagnosis of OMG.

* Corticosteroids might reduce the rate of generalization of OMG but remains controversial.

Bibliography

Chavis PS, Stickler DE, Walker A. Immunosuppressive or surgical treatment for ocular myasthenia gravis. *Arch Neurol.* 2007;64:1792-1794.

Gilbert ME, De Sousa EA, Savino PJ. Ocular myasthenia gravis treatment: the case against prednisone treatment. *Arch Neurol.* 2007;64:1790-1792.

Grob D. The course of MG and therapies affecting outcome. *Ann N Y Acad Sci.* 1987;505:472-499.

Kupersmith MJ, Latkany R, Homel P. Development of generalized disease at 2 years in patients with ocular myasthenia. *Arch Neurol.* 2003;60:243-248.

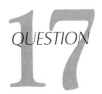

HOW DO YOU MANAGE VISUAL LOSS IN THYROID EYE DISEASE?

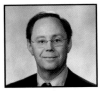

James A. Garrity, MD

A 50-year-old man with thyroid eye disease (TED) and long-standing diplopia and proptosis has recently noted progressive visual loss in one eye. The clinical exam suggests optic nerve dysfunction as the cause of diminished vision. How is the diagnosis of thyroid optic neuropathy established? What are the treatment options? How urgently should this patient be evaluated? When does the patient with TED require surgery? What surgeries are warranted and how urgently?

TED usually arises in the setting of Graves' disease with hyperthyroidism. From the ophthalmologist's perspective, thyroid status can be determined with 3 blood tests: 1) total T4, 2) thyroid-stimulating hormone (TSH), and 3) thyroid-stimulating immunoglobulins (TSI). Additional tests can be ordered, if needed, after discussing results of these tests with an endocrinologist. I expect that up to 90% of my patients with TED will be hyperthyroid but patients can be euthyroid or hypothyroid as well. The majority of TED patients in my practice, however, would be expected to have abnormal levels of TSI and a normal TSI should be a red flag in patients with the diagnosis of TED.

There are many potential causes of visual loss for your patient in the setting of TED. From a practical standpoint, however, you really should determine if the cornea or the optic nerve is responsible. It is important to differentiate the 2 causes since the treatment of each is vastly different.

In most cases of cornea-related visual loss, one would expect to find lid retraction with or without lagophthalmos. A more insidious cause is related to stiff eyelids with poor blinks. The eyelids do not close completely with blinks, leaving an interpalpebral zone (which includes the visual axis) of punctate keratopathy. Rose Bengal or fluorescein dye will highlight the area of involvement and lead to the correct diagnosis. Treatment is directed at better lubrication or in some instances eyelid surgery.

Vision loss related to optic neuropathy is typically insidious; a "sudden" onset is distinctly uncommon and in fact should prompt a search for a different diagnosis if this occurs. Did your patient suddenly "become aware" of reduced vision in one eye? This occurs typically when covering his or her good eye, which may account for some instances of "sudden" onset visual loss. In the setting of TED optic neuropathy (TEDON), the subjective perception is that the vision appears dim and colors may appear washed out. Objectively, visual acuity may be reduced, often to profound levels. On the other hand, visual acuity may remain normal with disc edema and/or visual field loss as the only findings. The examination should record visual acuity and a careful note of the pupillary responses. An afferent pupillary defect may not be present if the optic neuropathy is symmetric. Color vision is typically impaired. The external examination is surprising in that, many times, the eyes appear relatively white and quiet. Ocular motility is usually impaired to some degree, which is reflective of the underlying extraocular myopathy ultimately responsible for the optic neuropathy. Exceptionally, an optic neuropathy may not be compressive but rather can occur on the basis of a stretched optic nerve related to excessive proptosis from an expanded orbital fat compartment. As a general rule, patients with optic neuropathy tend to have less proptosis than patients without optic neuropathy, which may reflect a relative physiologic "auto-decompression" with excess proptosis in the nonoptic neuropathy group. The fundus examination may be entirely normal but approximately 30% of optic neuropathy patients have a swollen disc. Choroidal folds may also be present. Visual field examinations tend to show generalized depression, a central defect, or some type of an inferior defect. Any type of a superior defect should prompt a search for a different diagnosis. Imaging can be done with either magnetic resonance imaging (MRI) or computed tomography (CT); however, CT is my preference because bony details are shown. Appreciation of bony details is important if orbital decompression is a consideration.

I would not typically image the patient if I did not plan a decompression, but I would image if the TED was asymmetric enough to question the diagnosis or if there was some other atypical feature. The expected finding is apical compression from enlarged extraocular muscles. Iodine contrast is not needed as orbital fat serves as an inherent contrast. The iodine in the contrast also interferes with the endocrinologist's treatment of hyperthyroidism for at least 6 weeks. I do not see a role for visual evoked potentials in establishing the diagnosis of TEDON. While the diagnosis of TEDON was formerly considered an indication for emergent therapy, I am of the opinion that urgent therapy is soon enough. When I reviewed all the charts for our study of 215 patients with TEDON, it was apparent that many patients had their disease for many months and following therapy, their outcome was no different. Therefore, I have changed my approach in that therapy within the following few weeks was sufficient.

With an established diagnosis of TEDON the next question is what is the natural history of the disease? Does treatment favorably influence the course of the disease? There is limited data but Trobe et al did show that treatment was more effective than the natural history. Treatment is either nonsurgical or surgical. Nonsurgical therapy is centered on the use of corticosteroids. Steroids are effective although relapse and side effects limit their effectiveness. Co-morbid conditions such as diabetes also limit effectiveness of steroids. Rapamycin and cyclosporine have been utilized but treatment numbers are small. Radiation therapy also has limited experience. The reports of radiation therapy have the confounding variable of concomitant steroid use. Many patients with TEDON also have diabetes, which limits the use of radiation therapy because of the concern of radiation retinopathy. My treatment strategy has been to consider orbital decompression (transantral) as first line therapy with prolonged postoperative steroids as necessary. Decompression is associated with more rapid return of visual function, a median of 2.5 weeks in some series. I have used transfrontal decompression as salvage therapy for persistent TEDON. The group from Amsterdam, in a randomized clinical trial, showed that intravenous steroids were a better form of treatment than decompression. The trial had small numbers however.

Summary

* Patients with optic neuropathy make up a small but important segment of the TED practice.

* Noncontrast orbital CT scan might show the compressive optic neuropathy in TED and is also potentially useful for atypical cases due to alternative etiologies that might mimic TED (eg, sphenoid wing meningioma).

* There are many treatment options available for your patient and individualizing them is appropriate.

Bibliography

Fatourechi V, Bartley GB, Garrity JA, et al. Transfrontal orbital decompression after failure of transantral decompression in optic neuropathy of Graves' disease. *Mayo Clin Proc.* 1993;68:552-555.

Garrity JA, Fatourechi V, Bergstralh EJ, et al. Results of transantral orbital decompression in 428 patients with severe Graves' ophthalmopathy. *Am J Ophthalmol.* 1993;116:533-547.

Soares-Welch CV, Fatourechi V, Bartley GB, et al. Optic neuropathy of Graves' disease: results of transantral orbital decompression and long-term follow-up in 215 patients. *Am J Ophthalmol.* 2003;136:433-441.

Trobe JD, Glaser JS, Laflamme P. Dysthyroid optic neuropathy: clinical profile and rationale for management. *Arch Ophthalmol.* 1978;96:1199-1209.

Wakelkamp IMMJ, Baldeschi L, Saeed P, et al. Surgical or medical decompression as a first-line treatment of optic neuropathy in Graves' ophthalmopathy? A randomized controlled trial. *Clin Endocrinol.* 2005;63:323-328.

WHEN DO YOU USE RADIATION OR STEROIDS IN THYROID EYE DISEASE?

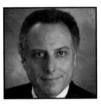

Steven E. Feldon, MD, MBA

A 56-year-old woman who is known to have thyroid eye disease (TED) for 6 months is being evaluated. Her vision has been stable, but she complains of significant eye swelling, tearing, and eye pain. She has no ophthalmoplegia, diplopia, or compressive optic neuropathy. Is there a role for corticosteroids in this patient's treatment? What about radiation therapy or surgery?

Determining the appropriate treatment for TED is complex and, in large part, governed by the intended goals of therapy, which can be either symptomatic relief alone or relief associated with compensation for physical changes occurring as part of the disease process. Making rational choices among treatment alternatives requires some understanding of the underlying disease process, including risk factors, pathology, and natural history.

Clinically significant TED occurs in about half of the patients with Graves' disease, and in 80% of cases, the onset is within a few months from the time the hyperthyroid state develops. Though hyperthyroidism is the largest risk factor for TED, smoking, age >50, hypertension, diabetes mellitus, and male gender are all associated with the disease. If any of these risk factors (such as abnormal thyroid hormone level, smoking, increased blood pressure, or increased blood sugar) are present in your patient, I suggest that they should be controlled as essential parts of managing her disease.

TED is characterized by mild symptoms such as ocular irritation, with resultant redness and tearing, as well as more substantial ones such as blurred vision, stare, double vision, and visual loss. These symptoms arise from an orbital inflammatory process that includes round cell infiltration, fibroblast proliferation, hyaluronic acid deposition, interstitial edema, and fat accumulation. The early tissue changes are likely the result of

Figure 18-1. Rundle's curve.

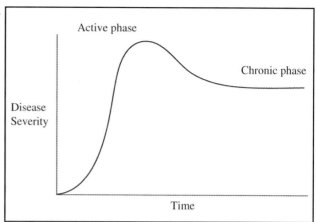

an autoimmune response precipitated by autoantigen presentation on some orbital cell types. Once the inflammation begins, other conditions may occur that result in secondary inflammation of the orbital tissues. These conditions are associated with the closed compartment formed by the bony orbit—processes such as venous stasis, capillary non-perfusion, and compression of soft tissues (eg, optic nerve).

Direct management of TED is constrained by 2 observations. The first observation is that the orbital inflammatory process is self-limited, progressing over 6 months to 3 years, with most progression noted in the first 18 months. This is sometimes called Rundle's curve. The second observation is that no medical treatment to date has proven highly efficacious in preventing onset of disease or in reversing the symptoms and signs.

With this background, your patient's treatment plan can be addressed. Her complaints suggest the presence of mild to moderate disease without marked muscle involvement. According to Rundle's curve (Figure 18-1), this patient has the potential for progressing but may also be entering a period of stability or even resolution. If this patient is still smoking, hyperthyroid, hypertensive, or hyperglycemic, these risk factors require immediate attention. This being stated, her symptoms are primarily related to fluid accumulation, dry eye, and possibly exposure. Thus, symptomatic relief can be achieved by addressing each of these processes. Fluid accumulation may be secondary to active inflammation, but venous stasis is a more likely cause. Elevating the head of the bed at night and using a mild diuretic often produce dramatic improvement. Frequent use of artificial tears or placement of punctual plugs alleviates much of the redness and tearing associated with dry eye. Rarely have I found topical corticosteroid application of value in reducing surface-related symptoms. Exposure secondary to upper and/or lower lid retraction with lagophthalmos can be addressed by taping the lids closed at night, which is preferable to ointments that provide protection for only a few hours. These simple steps, combined with the reassurance that her disease is likely close to stabilizing, are usually sufficient. Of course, once stability has been achieved, the patient may be concerned by appearance changes. These should be addressed surgically.

The use of corticosteroids or radiation therapy has not even been considered as yet. The rationale for intervention with these modalities assumes that the symptoms are due to active inflammatory disease activity and that the symptoms, left untreated, would progress or fail to resolve. As stated previously, these assumptions about disease activity may not be true. Markers for disease activity are highly controversial. They include the level of thyroid-binding immunoglobulins or other circulating factors as well as the presence of one or more symptoms or signs. Correlation of disease progression with circulating antibody levels has been poor. The use of symptoms or signs as a marker is flawed as both a tautology and an inappropriate assumption that inflammation is autoimmune rather than secondary due to tissue alterations.

Of course, if corticosteroids or radiation therapy are used, the perceived effect is likely to be indistinguishable from stabilization associated with Rundle's curve. Remember that transient improvement from corticosteroid use is likely from nonspecific reduction in inflammation. Similar results could have been obtained using previously described, conservative measures. This point of view is supported by the observation that tapering of corticosteroids is often associated with recurrence of symptoms and, therefore, steroid dependency. Several studies support the increased efficacy of high-dose, intravenous steroids. However, severe complications, including liver damage and death, have been reported. Orbital injection of corticosteroids has been utilized occasionally and is promoted by a few. While this modality usually spares the systemic manifestations of steroid use, potential local complications are substantial and include elevation of intraocular pressure; hemorrhage or inflammation associated with injections into a "tight," inflamed orbit; and granuloma formation. Since radiation is usually given with corticosteroids, the radiation effect is especially difficult to quantify. A prospective, masked study of the isolated effects of radiation therapy performed at Mayo Clinic failed to show any benefit, though the inclusion criteria preclude this study from being definitive in cases of recent-onset disease.

Summary

* Corticosteroids and radiation therapy are almost never indicated in mild to moderate TED.

* Surgical orbital decompression may be necessary for TED with optic nerve compression.

* Simple measures and reassurance will hopefully allow your patient to land safely on the plateau of Rundle's curve.

* Surgical reconstruction can be considered for functional and cosmetic indications once the patient is stable.

Bibliography

Bahn RS, Heufelder AE. Pathogenesis of thyroid eye disease. *N Engl J Med.* 1993;329:1468-1475.
Bartalena L, Marcocci C, Bogazzi F, Bruno-Bossio G, Pinchera A. Glucocorticoid therapy of Graves' ophthalmopathy. *Exp Clin Endocrinol.* 1991;97:320-327.
Gorman CA, Garrity JA, Fatoureschi V, et al. A prospective, double-blind, placebo-controlled study. *Lancet.* 2001; 355:1505-1509.
Prabhaker SB, Bahn RS, Smith J. Current perspective on the pathogenesis of Graves' disease and ophthalmopathy. *End Rev.* 2003;6:802-835.

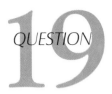
HOW DO YOU MANAGE
DIPLOPIA IN THYROID EYE DISEASE?

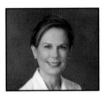

Kimberly Cockerham, MD

A 35-year-old woman with thyroid eye disease (TED) complains of worsening diplopia over the last several months. On examination she has mild proptosis, a small angle left hypertropia but a new exotropia.

Before delving into ophthalmology core history and physical, I am concerned that an exotropia is not typical for TED and so you need to search for evidence of myasthenia gravis or some other process coexisting with the TED.

It is important to ask if there are there are symptoms or signs of myasthenia gravis. Symptoms suggestive of myasthenia include the following:

* Double vision worse at the end of the day or with use (eg, computer work, reading, watching television)
* Ptosis of one or both eyelids that is worse at the end of the day or with use
* Afternoon tearing due to orbicularis weakness resulting in ectropion of puncta and/or eyelid
* Snarl appearance to mouth due to weak perioral muscles
* Weakness of proximal limbs causing difficulty climbing stairs or brushing hair
* Change in voice (nasal sounding)
* Difficulty swallowing or choking with normal bites of food
* Shortness of breath

It is especially important to note whether the patient's eyelids and eye position are variable or stable from hour to hour and day to day. Decreased visual acuity may indicate optic nerve or corneal compromise and can result in decreased vision that prompts sensory exotropia in patients without significant medial rectus restriction. Remember, TED characteristically enlarges and then restricts extraocular muscle activity, but some patients have minimal muscle enlargement and primarily intraconal fat expansion.

Ask your patient if his or her double vision is worse in the morning, mid-day, or evening. TED causes double vision that is worse in the morning whereas myasthenia gravis characteristically is associated with double vision that is worse at the end of the day. Both disorders are variable from hour to hour, day to day, and week to week. Both diseases result in double vision that is exacerbated with visual activities such as reading, working on the computer, and driving.

Remember, both TED and myasthenia can mimic a cranial nerve pattern of deviation, especially fourth and sixth nerve palsies. Of note, TED does not alter the velocity or accuracy of the saccade. In contrast, myasthenia gravis causes intrasaccadic delay and cranial nerve palsies are characterized by slowed saccades. Do not be confused if the deviation maps out to a fourth nerve palsy with a specific head tilt preference; this is widely reported. Isolated inferior oblique dysfunction has also been described.

TED typically causes elevation of the upper eyelids that is most pronounced laterally due to the fibers of Müller's muscle that extend between the orbital and palpebral lobes of the lacrimal gland. Any patient with drooping of the upper eyelid has myasthenia gravis until proven otherwise. Important historical points include variable ptosis that is worse in the evening or with activity, afternoon ectropion due to orbicularis weakness, and symptoms of proximal muscle weakness (new difficulty climbing stairs or brushing their hair, shortness of breath, and change in voice [nasalization], or ability to swallow [especially following prolonged chewing]).

I would suggest an ophthalmology examination focused on TED, but also look for signs of myasthenia gravis and other conditions that can mimic TED. This exam should include assessment of acuity, visual fields, and color vision. I feel that red desaturation is a terrific first sign in asymmetric TED optic nerve compression. Color plate testing and light brightness desaturation are also good. The afferent pupillary defect may be subtle in bilateral asymmetric cases. Proptosis quantification with Hertel's exophthalmometer is helpful, but subjective observation from above and below is essential in cases of subtle asymmetry. Resistance to retropulsion should be assessed. Firm pressure with the fingers from behind or thumbs from in front of the patient can be very helpful in establishing concern that an orbital process is occurring. Periorbital signs of active disease should also be assessed and include tenderness (and subjective pain/ache/pressure), redness, and edema that is worse in the morning. A pink caruncle is particularly characteristic. A lateral "fat pad" is often evident, giving the upper eyelid a "W" sign that looks as though there is a lateral fat pad in the upper eyelid (really the lacrimal gland prolapsed forward) and the lower eyelid (lateral fat prolapse both exacerbated by intraconal fat expansion).

The exam also needs to assess eyelid position and dynamics. The upper eyelid assumes a staring appearance during the active phase of hyperthyroidism and less commonly in other disorders of thyroid function. Lid lag is the dynamic reduction in descent velocity of the eyelid in attempted closure. This contrasts with lagophthalmos, which represents the separation in millimeters of the eyelids in passive downgaze. Test orbicularis strength

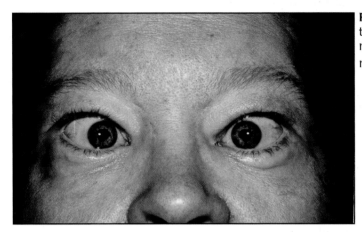

Figure 19-1. Vertical diplopia to restriction of upgaze is common as is esotropia due to medial rectus involvement.

by having the patient squeeze his or her eyes close and then look in same way as done to confirm Bell's phenomenon (upward deviation of eye with forced closure). Look for ptosis by quantitating the vertical palpebral fissure, the levator function, and the distance of the upper and lower eyelids from the corneal reflex.

The double vision of TED is typically due to inflammation and later restriction of the extraocular muscles. Vertical diplopia to restriction of upgaze is common as is esotropia due to medial rectus involvement as demonstrated in Figure 19-1.

I would then proceed with ancillary testing focused on TED (and myasthenia gravis). If ptosis is present, proceed with ice/rest test, sustained upgaze assessment (inability to maintain upgaze for 5 seconds), and Cogan's lid twitch testing (upward rebound of eyelid after sustained upgaze immediately followed by downgaze). If dysmotility is present, proceed with assessment of saccadic accuracy and velocity (Myasthenia gravis is characterized by intrasaccadic delay = fast then slowed saccades and a variety of other deviations from normal saccadic velocity and accuracy that are typical of TED). Visual fields should be performed at least once a year and whenever visual acuity is not corrected to 20/20 (without explanation). I find orbital ultrasound, if available, to be very helpful to demonstrate the enlarged extraocular muscles without tendon involvement or scleritis. Laboratory assessment should include thyroid-stimulating hormone (TSH), thyroid-stimulating immunoglobulin (TSI), and other standard thyroid function testing. For those with suspected myasthenia gravis, order the myasthenia gravis panel at your hospital, which includes acetylcholine receptor (ACHR) binding, blocking, and modulating antibodies. Less than 40% of patients with myasthenia gravis limited to the eyes demonstrate serum abnormalities. A Tensilon test should be performed if negative. Other ancillary testing such as single-fiber EMG testing can occasionally be diagnostic.

Once the inflammatory process is initiated in the orbital and periorbital tissues, normalization of thyroid function does not necessarily result in clinical improvement of TED. Worsening diplopia can definitely occur despite long-standing stable thyroid function. This does not mean thyroid function tests have no role in the management of TED. Patients with unstable thyroid function tests (TFTs), especially prolonged hypothyroidism, often have difficult-to-control TED.

Unless you have a strong suspicion that something else is going on in the orbit and there may be intracranial extension, get a computed tomography (CT) scan of the orbits with no contrast. The CT typically demonstrates enlargement of the extraocular muscles especially the medial and inferior rectus muscles with sparing of the tendons.

Summary

* In TED, an exotropia is *very* unusual and should warrant careful examination for coexisting myasthenia gravis.

* Myasthenia gravis occurs in at least 5% of patients with Graves' disease, so it should always be considered in patients with double vision that is worse at the end of the day or in patients with exotropia or ptosis.

* Imaging studies—both CT and MRI—should be carefully evaluated for another process such as lymphoma that happens to be occurring in conjunction with Graves' disease.

Bibliography

Dolman PJ, Rootman J. VISA classification for Graves's orbitopathy. *Ophthalmic Plast Reconstr Surg.* 2006;22:319-324.

Garrity JA, Bahn RS. Pathogenesis of graves ophthalmopathy: implications for prediction, prevention, and treatment. *Am J Ophthalmol.* 2006;142:147-153.

Hatton MP, Rubin PA. Controversies in thyroid-related orbitopathy: radiation and decompression. *Int Ophthalmol Clin.* 2005;45:1-14.

Krassas GE, Boboridis K. Recent developments in the medical treatment of thyroid eye disease. *Orbit.* 2006;25:117-122.

Peele KA, Kennerdell JS. *AAO, Focal Points: Thyroid-Associated Orbitopathy.* Module #1; 1997.

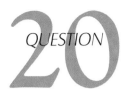
ARE THERE ANY TREATMENTS FOR NYSTAGMUS THAT WORK?

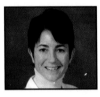

Janet C. Rucker, MD

The patient is a 35-year-old woman who has a long history of multiple sclerosis (MS). She complains of oscillopsia and is found to have pendular nystagmus. Can anything be offered to alleviate her nystagmus? Are there any treatments for nystagmus that actually work?

MS is a very common cause of acquired pendular nystagmus (APN), so from a diagnostic standpoint, it is very likely that your patient's nystagmus is directly attributable to the MS and alternative diagnostic testing would not generally be needed. I would, however, treat the onset of this new visual symptom as any other acute MS exacerbation and would obtain an updated magnetic resonance imaging (MRI) of the brain with gadolinium to look for active MS lesions (lesions demonstrating enhancement with gadolinium). Since vision loss can directly cause pendular nystagmus, I would also carefully assess for evidence of optic neuritis. As in any other acute MS exacerbation, I would discuss with the patient the potential benefit of a 3-day course of intravenous methylprednisolone (1 g/day) followed by a 2-week oral prednisone course, especially if other neurologic symptoms, such as gait deterioration, accompany the onset of oscillopsia. This having been said, APN in MS is often insidious and persistent, thereby requiring ongoing therapy to directly treat the visual consequences of APN. Unfortunately, it is one of the most visually disabling nystagmus waveforms.

The mainstay of therapy is pharmacologic and several good options exist for APN treatment. Gabapentin has a very tolerable side effect profile, a large dosing range, and its beneficial effects in suppressing oscillopsia and dampening the nys-

n APN have been demonstrated in a double-blind controlled
sons, my first treatment preference for your patient is gabapen-
fizer, New York, NY) (non-Food and Drug Administration [FDA]
Assuming normal renal function (impairment of which requires
the initial dose would be 300 mg of gabapentin 3 times a day. If
you   .elt too drowsy on this dose, the dose could be decreased to 100 mg
3 times a   . The dose should then be gradually increased by 300 mg every week or two
and her subjective response, visual acuity, and quantitative ocular motility recordings (if
available) reassessed after several weeks of therapy. I would continue to slowly titrate the
dose up to 1 of 3 endpoints: 1) development of intolerable side effects (drowsiness being
the most common), 2) visual benefit (at which point I would maintain the current dose),
or 3) a maximum dose of 1200 mg 3 times a day. If gabapentin is ineffective or incompletely effective when the endpoint is reached, I would add or change to a second agent.

My second medication preference for APN is memantine (Namenda, Forest
Pharmaceuticals, Inc, New York, NY) (non-FDA approved use). This is a weak N-
methyl-D-aspartate (NMDA) glutamate antagonist, approved in this country for the
treatment of Alzheimer's disease. It has been shown in a small case series of patients
to suppress the oscillations of APN. It should not be utilized in combination with
amantadine, which many MS patients take for fatigue. If the patient is on amantadine,
this should be discontinued prior to beginning therapy with memantine. The initial
starting dose of memantine is 5 mg daily, which is then slowly escalated by 5 mg per
week in twice-a-day dosing (5 mg twice a day for 1 week, then 10 mg in the morning,
and 5 mg at night for 1 week), to a maximum dose of 10 mg twice a day. This is the
maximum FDA-recommended dose for Alzheimer's disease; however, doses up to 20
mg twice daily have been safely used in other countries. If ineffective, I would taper
your patient off of memantine and give her a trial of clonazepam, starting at a dose of
1.5 mg daily in 3 divided doses. This could be slowly titrated to a maximum dose of
20 mg daily in divided doses. This treatment option is less well supported in the literature, but clonazepam (Klonopin, Roche, Nutley, NJ) is anecdotally effective in treating
many nystagmus types. Baclofen (Lioresal, Novartis, New York, NY) may be tried but was
ineffective in suppressing APN in a trial comparing gabapentin to baclofen.

Although extraocular muscle surgical options are generally reserved for congenital
nystagmus, there are some recent published cases demonstrating improvement in APN
in MS patients following surgical intervention. Most of these patients had APN that was
unresponsive (or only partially responsive) to medical therapy (usually with gabapentin
or memantine) and most had an ocular misalignment (internuclear ophthalmoplegia
with exotropia or cranial nerve palsy) in addition to the nystagmus. The surgeries tend
to incorporate both "nystagmus surgery" (usually utilizing tenotomy) and traditional
strabismus surgery for the correction of the ocular deviation. This may be attempted for
intractable and visually disabling APN when medical therapy alone is incompletely effective, although guidance is purely anecdotal.

Two additional therapeutic options are optical therapy with prisms and botulinum
toxin. If her nystagmus is dampened with ocular convergence, base-out prisms may be
tried; whereas base-in prisms may be tried if the nystagmus increases with convergence.
Several anecdotal beneficial responses to retrobulbar botulinum toxin injection are
reported in patients with acquired nystagmus. The effect tends to last for 1 to 3 months.

While some patients have transient or no side effects, others are so significantly bothered by diplopia and ptosis that they elect not to undergo repeat injection.

Summary

* MS is a very common cause of APN.
* The main pharmacologic options for APN treatment include gabapentin and memantine, and perhaps clonazepam or baclofen.

Bibliography

Averbuch-Heller L, Tusa RJ, Fuhry L, et al. A double-blind controlled study of gabapentin and baclofen as treatment for acquired nystagmus. *Ann Neurol.* 1997;41:818-825.

Jain S, Proudlock F, Constantinescu CS, Gottlob I. Combined pharmacologic and surgical approach to acquired nystagmus due to multiple sclerosis. *Am J Ophthalmol.* 2002;134:780-782.

Starck M, Albrecht H, Pollman W, Straube A, Dieterich M. Drug therapy for acquired pendular nystagmus in multiple sclerosis. *J Neurol.* 1997;244:9-16.

Tomsak RL, Dell'Osso LF, Rucker JC, Leigh RJ, Bienfang DC, Jacobs JB. Treatment of acquired pendular nystagmus from multiple sclerosis with eye muscle surgery followed by oral memantine. *Dig J Ophthalmol.* 2006;11:1-11.

HOW DO YOU EVALUATE DOWNBEAT NYSTAGMUS?

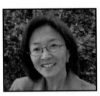

Sophia M. Chung, MD

A 56-year-old woman who is found to have downbeat nystagmus is being evaluated. What are the possible causes? What work-up should be instituted? What if a magnetic resonance imaging (MRI) shows no structural lesion of the cerebellum or brainstem?

Downbeat nystagmus is rhythmic vertical oscillations with the fast phase in the downward direction. The movements increase in amplitude and frequency in lateral gaze just below midline. They may also increase in downgaze but dampen in upgaze in as many as 45% of patients. In patients with downbeat nystagmus, the eyes are expected to show an upward slow-phase with a corrective downward fast-phase in primary position. Sometimes, magnification is required either by slit lamp examination or funduscopy. Characteristically, this form of nystagmus increases in amplitude and frequency on lateral gaze and often in downgaze. The nystagmus may dampen, persist, or change direction in upgaze. Patients with downbeat nystagmus are often aware that the oscillopsia or blurred vision increases with right and left gaze and may recognize depression of the chin improves vision as the nystagmus may show a null zone where the nystagmus is abolished or quietest. Sometimes, however, the downbeat nystagmus may be unchanged in upgaze or switch direction to an upbeat nystagmus.

In your patient, I would be concerned about the most common cause for downbeat nystagmus, a disease process affecting the cervicomedullary junction. Arnold-Chiari malformations and both hereditary and sporadic spinocerebellar degenerations account for the majority of downbeat nystagmus. However, other causes include infarction, multiple sclerosis, tumors in the posterior fossa, rarely hydrocephalus, and drug toxicities.

Lithium, alcohol, phenytoin, carbamazepine, and morphine intoxication have all been reported to cause downbeat nystagmus. Conversely, deficiencies of magnesium and B_{12} particularly in patients with gastrointestinal disease can cause this finding. Downbeat nystagmus may rarely occur as a paraneoplastic phenomenon. Breast, ovarian, and lung carcinomas are the most commonly associated tumors. A few patients have been found to have encephalitis as the mechanism of their downbeat nystagmus. However, 40% to 50% of patients do not have an identifiable cause despite detailed neurologic and radiologic investigations.

I would ask your patient about the onset of symptoms (abrupt, gradual), their duration, whether the symptoms are constant versus intermittent, and about any associated signs or symptoms particularly neurologic in nature. A medical history for prior stroke, multiple sclerosis, head trauma, bipolar disease, or other health conditions requiring medications is critical. A social history investigating alcohol intake and nutritional habits is similarly important. I would suggest that your patient be examined by a neurologist for accompanying signs of neurologic disease such as ataxia, dysarthria, or localizing signs.

Beyond the office, the first test of choice is an MRI of the brain with gadolinium with special attention to the posterior fossa. Herniation of the cerebellar tonsils, brainstem and/or cerebellar stroke, demyelinating disease, and tumors should be ruled out. Atrophy of the cerebellum and/or brainstem is consistent with spinocerebellar degenerations but is not required for the diagnosis. If there is no identifiable disease on MRI, laboratory investigations should include levels for medications when applicable, B_{12}, and magnesium levels. Levels for drugs need not be the "toxic" range defined by the laboratory to cause nystagmus and the drug may need to be discontinued to determine toxicity. Chronic lithium ingestion may cause irreversible downbeat nystagmus despite discontinuation of the drug. Paraneoplastic disease should be ruled out as well. A paraneoplastic antibody panel may be drawn but patients should be counseled to have updated breast and pelvic examinations, mammograms, and—where applicable—a chest x-ray and/or computed tomography (CT) of the chest. Finally, some patients may require spinal fluid analysis to rule out demyelinating disease or encephalitis.

The treatment lies with reversing the primary identifiable cause or instituting appropriate management. In patients with Arnold-Chiari malformation, suboccipital decompression can reverse or dampen the nystagmus but not always. Patients suffering from drug intoxication should be withdrawn from the offending agent or the dose lowered. Conversely, deficiencies of magnesium, thiamine, or B_{12} should be appropriately corrected. Patients with tumors must seek neurosurgical, oncological, and radiation oncology consultations for appropriate management. Neurologic diseases such as spinocerebellar atrophy, multiple sclerosis, stroke, paraneoplastic disease, and encephalitis likewise must be evaluated and properly managed.

In as many as half of the patients, however, an etiology for the downbeat nystagmus is not identified. Also, treatment of the underlying condition may fail to adequately control their nystagmus and symptoms. What can we offer these patients? A variety of medications have been used to dampen if not abolish the nystagmus. Clonazepam, diazepam, and baclofen have been used with generally poor success and are complicated by the sedating effects. Gabapentin has been used with considerably better success although less effective for vertical nystagmus than horizontal. More recently, 3,4 diaminopyridine and 4-aminopyridine, potassium channel blockers, have shown conflicting results in affecting downbeat nystagmus. These medications are thought to enhance Purkinje cell activity, allowing restoration of inhibition of vertical eye movements. Optical treatment modalities include use of single focus readers with instruction to raise the reading materials into the field of least movement, vertical prisms to deflect the images into the null zone, and base-out prisms to induce convergence as a small number of patients exhibit dampening with convergence. Unfortunately, the majority of patients with downbeat nystagmus exhibit increased amplitude and frequency on convergence. A surgical option includes Kestenbaum-Anderson–type procedures moving the vertical recti such that the null zone is moved inferiorly and therefore allowing improved visual function in primary position and in downgaze. Botulinum toxin has been used in selected patients with nystagmus but the patients must be well informed of the limited period of action, severe ophthalmoplegia, and need to view monocularly.

Summary

* Downbeat nystagmus is an important sign of potentially serious neurologic disease, especially affecting the cervicomedullary junction, and warrants a detailed neuro-ophthalmologic and neurologic examination.

* Many patients with downbeat nystagmus harbor tumors or neurodegenerative disease while others have readily reversible conditions such as nutritional deficiencies or drug toxicities.

* Patients with downbeat nystagmus require neuroradiologic investigation, preferably with an MRI with gadolinium, and likely will also require additional laboratory investigations particularly if neuroimaging is unrevealing.

Bibliography

Averbuch-Heller L, Tusa RJ, Fuhry L, et al. A double-blind controlled study of gabapentin and baclofen as treatment for acquired nystagmus. *Ann Neurol.* 1997;41:818-825.

Dieterich M, Straube A, Brandt T, Paulus W, Buttner U. The effects of baclofen and cholinergic drugs on upbeat and downbeat nystagmus. *J Neurol Neurosurg Psychiatry.* 1991;54:627-632.

Halmagyi GM, Rudge P, Gresty MA, Snaders MD. Downbeating nystagmus: a review of 62 cases. *Arch Neurol.* 1983;40:777-784.

Schmidt D. Downbeat nystagmus: a clinical review. *Neuro-Ophthalmology.* 1991;11:247-262.

Yee RD. Downbeat nystagmus: characteristics and localization of lesions. *Trans Amer Ophthalmol Soc.* 1989;87: 984-1032.

WHAT IS THE EVALUATION FOR ANISOCORIA?

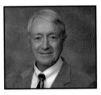

Brian R. Younge, MD

A 45-year-old woman who has anisocoria of unknown duration is being examined. In a patient with anisocoria, how do you decide if the big pupil or the small pupil is the problem?

The patient in question with incidental anisocoria of unknown duration presents an office challenge that can usually be resolved. Check to see if the anisocoria is greater in dim light and for the reaction of the pupils to light. If the anisocoria is greater in dim light (stimulates dilation of the normal pupil), then the defect is in the sympathetic innervation to the pupil. If the anisocoria is less in dim light, then the lesion is in the parasympathetic innervation to the pupil. Ptosis can accompany lesions of either pathway; it tends to be rather severe with third nerve lesions but is mild and certainly incomplete with lesions of the sympathetic pathway, which result in lack of tone of Müller's muscle.

In your patient, if the pupillary light reaction is normal in both eyes, then physiologic (simple) anisocoria, Horner syndrome, or sympathetic irritation should be considered.

Between 15% and 30% of the normal population have simple anisocoria with a difference in pupillary size of 0.4 mm or greater. These patients have no associated ptosis or dilation lag and no evidence of iris injury or topical drugs. Topical cocaine will dilate both pupils equally. If this is Horner syndrome, the anisocoria will become more pronounced when the lights in the examining room are turned off. While the lights are being turned off, one should look for a "dilatation lag" of the smaller pupil. If present, there may be more pupillary asymmetry 5 seconds after the lights are turned off than 15 seconds afterward. A dilatation lag implies poor sympathetic tone and is therefore indicative of Horner syndrome. Ask about things like headache or neck pain on the side of the smaller pupil (carotid dissection) or any recent surgical procedures in which a line might have been placed in the neck. If there is heterochromia, this may be congenital Horner syndrome. Ask the patient about sweating abnormalities in the face and hands. Drug tests are handy to discern the localization of a Horner's pupil, and if you are clinically certain, skip the cocaine test because it merely confirms what you already know. If you can get hydroxyamphetamine, use that as it helps to distinguish a Horner pupil due to the last neuron in the sympathetic chain from the central or intermediate neuron. If there is no dilation of the small pupil, but the other one dilates well and the lid stays down, the final neuron is involved, and this is almost always a more benign problem.

If anisocoria is present and one of the pupils, generally the larger one, reacts poorly to light, the diagnosis in your patient can be narrowed to 4 possibilities: 1) third nerve palsy, 2) tonic pupil, 3) iris damage, or 4) drug-induced anisocoria.

Patients with anisocoria and a poorly reactive pupil should be evaluated for an ipsilateral third nerve palsy. A young patient with a thunderclap headache and a dilated pupil on one side has an aneurysm until proven otherwise. Check the ocular motility for other signs of third nerve paresis. The pupil sign can be the first clue to an impending third nerve palsy and subarachnoid hemorrhage. Although an extra-axial lesion (eg, unruptured intracranial aneurysm) compressing the third nerve may extremely rarely cause a dilated pupil in isolation (or with minimal ocular motor nerve paresis), in the absence of an extraocular motility deficit and/or ptosis, an isolated dilated pupil is usually not due to third nerve paresis. If there are signs of motility impairment, suggesting a third nerve palsy, emergency neurologic evaluation and investigations in your patient are necessary.

Look at the pupil both grossly with a penlight and with slit lamp, looking for response to light, the near stimulus, and see if there is evidence of sector weakness, particularly in the more dilated pupil, as this could be a tonic (Adie's) pupil. With a tonic pupil, there is usually mydriasis with a poor or absent reaction to light but a slow constriction to prolonged near effort (light-near dissociation). Redilation after constriction to near stimuli is slow and tonic. Segmental vermiform movements of the iris borders may be evident on slit lamp exam (due to sector palsy of other areas of the iris sphincter), and cholinergic supersensitivity of the denervated iris sphincter (constriction when 0.1% pilocarpine is instilled) may be demonstrated. Tonic pupils occur from local damage to the ciliary ganglion or short ciliary nerves, as part of a widespread peripheral or autonomic neuropathy, or in otherwise healthy individuals (Adie's tonic pupil syndrome). With time, ciliary muscle dysfunction tends to resolve, and the pupil becomes progressively miotic ("little old Adie's"). Some patients may have primary miotic Adie's pupils without passing through a mydriatic phase. There is a tendency for patients with unilateral Adie's syndrome to develop a tonic pupil in the opposite eye.

Damage to the iris due to ischemia, trauma, or an inflammatory process may cause mydriasis. Clinical characteristics of suggesting abnormalities of the iris structure as a cause for mydriasis include no associated ptosis or ocular motility disturbance (versus third nerve palsy), the pupil is often irregular with tears in pupillary margin due to tears in iris sphincter (versus smooth margin in drug-related pupillary abnormalities), and irregular contraction of the pupil to light. The eventual development of iris atrophy may occur, and poor or no response of the pupil to 1% pilocarpine.

Mydriasis may be induced by the instillation of a parasympatholytic drug (eg, atropine, scopolamine). Someone who works with drugs like atropine or norepinephrine may get a little on the finger and subsequently rub the eye. Or the mom who is demonstrating to her little child how easy it is to take an eye drop (atropine) may have inadvertently contaminated her fingers and transferred it to her own eye. Unilateral mydriasis may follow the use of transdermal scopolamine to prevent motion sickness, the accidental instillation into the eye of fluids from certain plants (eg, jimsonweed) that contain belladonna and atropine-like alkaloids, and exposure to certain cosmetics and perfumes. A careful history is usually all that is required in patients with inadvertent or intentional (eg, glaucoma medication, treatment with topical cycloplegics for uveitis) exposure to agents that may affect pupil size.

Nurses, physicians, and other health care workers are particularly prone to inadvertent or intentional exposure to pharmacological mydriatics. The pupil size of patients with pharmacologic sphincter blockade is often quite large (>8 mm), often on the order of 10 to 12 mm in diameter, which is much greater than the mydriasis usually seen in a typical third nerve palsy or tonic pupil syndromes. The pupils are evenly affected 360 degrees (versus a tonic pupil) and smoothly affected around without irregularity (versus iris trauma). A solution of pilocarpine (1%) causes constriction in the case of a third nerve lesion but does not modify pupillary size if the anisocoria is due to an atropinic drug or to iris damage. Remember, however, that some patients with Adie's syndrome of recent onset may have a fixed dilated pupil that fails to constrict to even a strong solution of pilocarpine. Adrenergic pharmacologic mydriasis (eg, phenylephrine) may be clinically distinguished by blanched conjunctival vessels, residual light reaction, and a retracted upper lid due to sympathetic stimulation of the upper lid retractor muscle. With adrenergic mydriasis, the pupil may react to bright light due to the working iris sphincter muscle, which can overcome dilator spasm.

Summary

* If anisocoria is greater in dim light (stimulates dilation of the normal pupil), then the defect is in the sympathetic innervation to the pupil. If the anisocoria is greater in bright light, then the lesion is in the parasympathetic innervation to the pupil or iris.

* If the pupillary light reaction is normal in both eyes, then physiologic (simple) anisocoria, Horner syndrome, or sympathetic irritation should be considered.

* If anisocoria is present and one of the pupils, generally the larger one, reacts poorly to light, the diagnosis is narrowed to third nerve palsy, tonic pupil, iris damage, or drug-induced anisocoria.

* If anisocoria is associated with signs of motility impairment, suggesting a third nerve palsy, emergency neurologic evaluation and investigations are necessary.

Bibliography

Eggenberger, ER. DO: Anisocoria, in eMedicine Specialties

Lee AG, Brazis PW. *Clinical Pathways in Neuro-Ophthalmology: An Evidence-Based Approach.* 2nd ed. New York: Thieme; 2003.

Thompson HS, Corbett JJ, Kline LB, et al. Pseudo-Horner's syndrome. *Arch Neurol.* 1982;39:108-111.

Thompson HS, Pilley SFJ. Unequal pupils: a flow chart for sorting out the anisocorias. *Sum Ophthalmol.* 1976;21:45-48.

HOW AND WHEN SHOULD I WORK-UP HORNER SYNDROME?

Valérie Biousse, MD

A 55-year-old hypertensive man complains of acute headache on the left and is found to have a left Horner syndrome. What evaluation is necessary with Horner syndrome and how urgently should it be performed? Are there any life-threatening etiologies of a Horner syndrome?

This patient with an acute isolated painful Horner syndrome is considered to have a left internal carotid artery dissection until proven otherwise. He needs to be evaluated emergently in neurology with noninvasive vascular imaging. If a dissection is confirmed, he will need to be admitted and treated to prevent a cerebral infarction.

The diagnosis of Horner syndrome is most often easy just based on the findings of anisocoria, with the small pupil not dilating well in the dark and decreased ipsilateral palpebral fissure. Horner syndrome results from dysfunction of the ipsilateral sympathetic pathway and is also called oculosympathetic paresis. Signs of Horner syndrome include reduced palpebral fissure with mild ptosis involving both upper and lower lids due to paralysis of the Müller's muscles innervated by the sympathetic pathway, pseudo-enophthalmos because of the reduced palpebral fissure, unilateral miosis, dilation lag in the dark (slow dilation of the affected pupil), and heterochromia in congenital Horner syndrome (lighter color on affected side). Associated neurologic symptoms and signs such as anhidrosis of ipsilateral face may occur with preganglionic lesions (first or second order) while brainstem and spinal cord symptoms and signs suggest a first-order Horner syndrome. Associated arm pain, hand weakness, history of neck surgery, or neck trauma suggest a second-order Horner syndrome (Figure 23-1).

Figure 23-1. Right Horner syndrome. There is slight decrease of the palpebral fissure on the right and the right pupil is smaller than the left pupil.

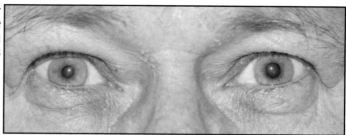

Figure 23-2. Diagnosis of Horner syndrome with apraclonidine drops (same patient as in Figure 23-1). The anisocoria is reversed with the right pupil being now slightly larger than the left pupil. The palpebral fissures are now symmetric.

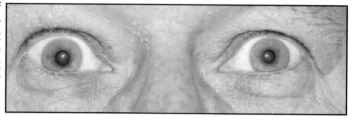

Pharmacological testing confirms the diagnosis of Horner syndrome in subtle cases.

Cocaine drops are most commonly used (but are now difficult to obtain). Apraclonidine drops (used for glaucoma; off-label application) are now replacing cocaine for the diagnosis of Horner syndrome because they are easy to obtain (Figure 23-2).

To perform a cocaine test, instill 2 drops of 4% or 10% cocaine in both eyes. Forty-five minutes to 1 hour later, a normal pupil dilates while the Horner pupil dilates poorly and the anisocoria increases. Cocaine blocks the reuptake of norepinephrine at the sympathetic nerve synapse with the iris dilator. It causes pupillary dilation in eyes with intact sympathetic innervation but has no effect in eyes with impaired sympathetic innervation, regardless of the lesion location (little or no norepinephrine is being released into the synaptic cleft tonically).

Testing with apraclonidine involves instillation of 2 drops of 0.5% or 1% apraclonidine in both eyes. After 30 to 45 minutes, a normal pupil does not dilate while a Horner pupil dilates and the anisocoria reverses. The palpebral fissure enlarges (apraclonidine reverses the Horner syndrome). Apraclonidine is a direct α-receptor agonist (strong α2 and weak α1). It has no effect in eyes with intact sympathetic innervation but causes mild pupillary dilation in eyes with sympathetic denervation regardless of the lesion location (with denervation hypersensitivity, α1 effect dilates the Horner pupil).

Horner syndrome may be caused by a lesion anywhere along the sympathetic pathway that supplies the head, eye, and neck. Associated symptoms and signs usually allow localization of the lesion.

When you see a patient with new anisocoria possibly related to a Horner syndrome, you have to decide whether to confirm the Horner pharmacologically (with cocaine or apraclonidine) or to localize the lesion along the sympathetic pathway with hydroxyamphetamine. When the diagnosis of Horner syndrome is obvious clinically, I prefer to immediately localize the lesion by performing a pharmacologic test with hydroxyamphetamine 1%. When testing with hydroxyamphetamine (off-label application of drug), instill 2 drops of 1% hydroxyamphetamine in both eyes. Forty-five minutes later a normal pupil dilates while a Horner pupil dilates poorly if the lesion is postganglionic (third order). The Horner pupil dilates if the lesion is preganglionic (first or second order). Hydroxyamphetamine releases stored norepinephrine from the postganglionic adrenergic nerve endings. It causes pupillary dilation in eyes with intact sympathetic innervation or intact postganglionic fibers, but it has no or partial effect in eyes with impaired sympathetic innervation from lesions involving the postganglionic fibers (no effect on third-order Horner).

Except for rare emergencies, pharmacologic localization of the lesion should ideally be performed before obtaining any neuroimaging in adults. The evaluation of an adult with Horner syndrome is mostly based on lesion location. The most classic cause of central (first-order neuron) Horner is a lateral medullary infarction (Wallenberg syndrome); other causes include various thalamic, brainstem, and spinal cord lesions. Second-order Horner syndromes are most suggestive of neoplasm or trauma of the lower cervical spine, brachial plexus, or lung apex. Third-order Horner syndromes point to lesions of the internal carotid artery such as dissection or cavernous sinus aneurysms. Further evaluation depends upon the duration of symptoms, the presence of pain, other symptoms or signs, and the localization of the lesion to the first- or second-order neuron or to the third-order neuron. The most common causes of Horner syndrome in adults based on lesion location are included in Table 23-1.

All patients need a physical examination (ocular, neurologic, neck, supraclavicular, chest). The tests ordered will vary depending on the lesion location, the presence of associated symptoms or signs, the urgency of the work-up, and the radiologist's preference. If a first- or second order Horner is present, I suggest computed tomography (CT) or magnetic resonance imaging (MRI) of the chest (to view pulmonary apex), MRI head and neck with contrast, and possibly a magnetic resonance angiography (MRA) of the aortic arch or CTA (CT angiogram) of the head and neck. If a third-order Horner is present, I suggest MRI of the head with contrast and MRA or CTA of the head and neck. If localization of the Horner syndrome is unknown, I suggest imaging the brain, neck, spinal cord, carotid arteries, and pulmonary apex (may require multiple imaging tests). I feel that in this situation that the easiest test is a CT/CTA of the head, neck, and chest, which allows good examination of the brain and spine; the soft tissues; and large blood vessels in the head, neck and chest; it also allows examination of the pulmonary apex. Some authorities suggest MRI and MRA of the head, neck, and pulmonary apex using predefined Horner protocols.

Pearls to remember include a combination of an ipsilateral Horner syndrome (first order) and contralateral superior oblique palsy (fourth nerve palsy) suggests a lesion of the trochlear nucleus or its fascicle in the brainstem; a combination of an ipsilateral Horner syndrome (third order) and an abducens paresis (sixth nerve palsy) suggests a lesion in the cavernous sinus; an acute painful Horner syndrome should be presumed related to a dissection of the ipsilateral internal carotid artery unless proven otherwise (these patients are at risk of cerebral infarction and should be evaluated emergently). In many patients, especially patients with a third-order Horner syndrome, no etiology may be discovered.

Most patients with Horner syndrome have no visual changes and tolerate a mild ptosis. Rarely, lid surgery is requested to correct a persistent ptosis. Topical apraclonidine corrects the ptosis associated with Horner syndrome and may be used intermittently for cosmetic reasons or when the ptosis reduces the superior visual field.

Table 23-1

Most Common Causes of Horner Syndrome in Adults Based on Lesion Location

Central (First Order)	*Preganglionic (Second Order)*	*Postganglionic (Third Order)*
Hypothalamus • Stroke • Tumor	**Cervical spine disease** **Brachial plexus injury**	**Superior cervical ganglion** • Trauma • Jugular venous ectasia • Iatrogenic (surgical neck dissection)
Brainstem • Stroke (lateral medullary infarction) • Demyelination • Tumor	**Pulmonary apical lesions** • Apical lung tumor • Mediastinal tumors • Cervical rib • Trauma • Iatrogenic (jugular cannulation, chest tube, thoracic surgery) **Subclavian artery aneurysm**	**Internal carotid artery** • Dissection • Aneurysm • Trauma • Arteritis • Tumor
Spinal cord (cervicothoracic) • Trauma • Syringomyelia • Tumor (intramedullary) • Demyelination • Myelitis • Arteriovenous malformation	**Thyroid tumors**	**Skull base lesions (nasopharyngeal carcinoma, lymphoma)** **Cavernous sinus lesion** • Tumors • Pituitary tumor • Inflammation • Thrombosis • Carotid aneurysm **Cluster headache**

Summary

* Although a diagnosis of Horner syndrome may simply be based on the findings of anisocoria, with the small pupil not dilating well in the dark and decreased ipsilateral palpebral fissure, often pharmacologic testing with cocaine or apraclonidine drops is necessary to confirm the diagnosis in subtle cases.

* If a first- or second-order Horner is present, a CT or MRI of the chest (to view pulmonary apex), MRI head and neck with contrast, and possibly an MRA of the aortic arch or CTA of the head and neck are suggested.

* If a third-order Horner is present, MRI of the head with contrast and MRA or CTA of the head and neck is suggested.

* If localization of the Horner syndrome is unknown, images of the brain, neck, spinal cord, carotid arteries, and pulmonary apex should be performed.

Bibliography

Kawasaki A. Disorders of pupillary function, accommodation, and lacrimation. In: Miller NR, Newman NJ, Biousse V, Kerrison JB, eds. *Walsh and Hoyt's Clinical Neuro-Ophthalmology.* 6th ed. Philadelphia, PA: Lippincott, Williams, and Wilkins; 2005:739-805.

Thompson HS. Diagnosing Horner's syndrome. *Trans Amer Acad Ophthalmol Otolaryngol.* 1977;83:840-842.

WHAT SHOULD I DO WITH
A DILATED PUPIL?

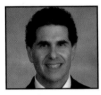

Randy Kardon, MD, PhD

A 44-year-old woman is being evaluated and the acute onset of a large pupil on the right side was noted. She is certain that it was not there 2 days ago. She is being seen 3 days after onset of the problem. The right pupil is 6 mm and nonreactive to light and near and the left pupil is 4 mm and reactive to light and near. Motility exam is completely normal. What are the possible etiologies for this abnormality? Could this still be an early third nerve palsy? Can any eyedrops help in the differential at this early time?

In the case above, it is stated that the right pupil is nonreactive to light or near effort and the fellow left pupil is normal in that it does react to both light and near. I usually use the spotlight in the exam lane over the exam chair to give as bright of light as possible to confirm that the anisocoria increases in bright light, revealing that the problem is in the right pupil, in this case.

The next big branching point of consideration of the etiology is to determine if the dilated nonreactive pupil is caused by iris sphincter palsy or excessive activation of the dilator muscle. Iris sphincter palsy is the more common. My first step is to establish that there is no associated motility disturbance, in particular, that this is an isolated mydriasis without extraocular motor signs of an oculomotor nerve palsy. Sometimes early involvement of the oculomotor nerve can be subtle and the patient may not be aware of diplopia or mild associated ptosis. Even if the patient has no symptoms of diplopia or shift on cross cover testing, I usually take the time to show him or her a penlight in extreme fields of gaze with a red filter held over one eye in order to make sure that there is not very mild, early oculomotor dysfunction. Once you have established that there is no misalignment even in extreme gaze, the chances are extremely rare that you are dealing with pupil involvement from early oculomotor nerve involvement. It is possible to have pupil involvement precede the extraocular involvement due to the medial location of the pupillary fibers along the intracranial course of the third nerve, but this is rare.

My next step is to determine if there is evidence for a segmental palsy. If the extraocular motility is normal, I then look carefully at the movement of the iris around the pupil border using the magnification of a slit lamp, turning on and off the slit lamp beam to observe whether there is any evidence for the presence of segmental palsy. The significance of a segmental nature to the palsy is important because it helps in localizing the lesion to the postganglionic territory. I have yet to observe an acute preganglionic efferent pupil defect that affected some segments of the iris sphincter and not others. I view segmental palsy with intervening, normally working sphincter segments as a sign of either a postganglionic parasympathetic lesion or direct damage to some segments of the iris sphincter muscle from ischemia. Yes, it is possible to damage all segments of the iris sphincter, but this is very rare and usually there is at least one small segment spared in the setting of postganglionic parasympathetic denervation or direct damage to the iris sphincter muscle. You should be watching one quadrant at a time while turning on and off the slit lamp beam. I look for some segments contracting in concert, while adjacent segments are sluggish, sometimes being pulled passively toward the clock hour where the sector is working normally. When an asymmetry is observed, it is very repeatable with each light stimulus. In some cases of segmental sphincter palsy, the cause is not denervation, but rather direct damage to the sphincter muscle from ischemia (either previous high intraocular pressure from angle closure or pigmentary dispersion, ocular ischemia, or iris vasculitis from Herpes zoster). My next step is to narrow the slit beam and direct it straight into the pupil to give a red reflex while turning up the intensity. I then look carefully for retroillumination defects in the iris as footprints of iris atrophy. Retroillumination defects in the iris tell me that there was probably direct damage to the iris sphincter muscle and not denervation. The presence or absence of segmental palsy or sparing of some areas of the iris sphincter can be even better seen with infrared iris transillumination.

Next, if the patient is still of an age where accommodative amplitude is still measurable (middle aged or younger), I make an effort to quantify his or her accommodative amplitude in each eye separately by measuring his or her near point of accommodation while he or she is wearing his or her distant correction. This tells you if the ciliary body is also affected either by denervation or by pharmacological influences. I measure this before and after any pharmacological testing, too. Keep in mind that anticholinergic ag__ nd parasympathetic nerve palsies will affect both the pupil and accommodation.
es, if the denervation is segmental and involves a sector of the ciliary body mus-
luced astigmatic error can also be present. In such cases, it is evident with a
and can be seen with retinoscopy as an induced cylinder refractive error with
tion. Another important but often under-appreciated sign: sympathomimet-
thetic discharge can also inhibit accommodative amplitude, but to a lesser
arasympathetic inhibition, usually in the order of 1 to 3 D. Most clinicians
sure accommodative amplitude, yet it is an important piece of information.
ften ask the patient how he or she discovered the unequal pupils, since the acute aspect is sometimes misleading. In other words, the patient may have acutely noticed it, but it may have been there awhile. Here, asking about light sensitivity or difficulty

focusing at near may help verify the timing of the event. Also, old pictures or even a magnified view of the patient's driver's license photo under the slit lamp can sometimes be revealing. If the cause is postganglionic parasympathetic denervation (eg, Adie's pupil) and it has been present for more than 2 months, then there should be some aspect of aberrant regeneration with light near dissociation on careful examination. Conversely, if the denervation is really acute, there should be no sign of light near dissociation. Another aspect to the evaluation that may be misleading is measuring the pupil diameter either directly or in photographs under different lighting conditions or with near response without taking into account a segmental aspect to the palsy. If a patient gives a good near effort, the unaffected segments may react enough to cause an overall decrease in diameter of the pupil, whereas a suboptimal light stimulus may produce a smaller diameter change, even though there is no real light near dissociation. So, it is very important to evaluate the segmental movement of the iris with bright light and near effort, in addition to documenting overall change in pupil size.

Pharmacologic mydriasis (from either anticholinergic or sympathomimetic agents) may be associated with some pupil reaction to light and near, especially if the contamination was weak or if the pharmacologic mydriasis is starting to wear off. In these cases, the pupil reaction is never segmental. The pupil may react some to direct-acting cholinergic stimulation (0.5% pilocarpine) but not as much as the control opposite eye 30 minutes after having received the same drop. If pharmacologic mydriasis is suspected, then I inform the patient that he or she should start to see it go away within the next few days (unless he or she is doing it intentionally). Sometimes, I have the patient take a digital picture in bright light at home in a few days and email it to me for confirmation.

Figure 24-1 demonstrates the clinical findings in a patient with an Adie's pupil.

Summary

* In a patient with unilateral mydriasis, first demonstrate that it is isolated, without any accompanying extraocular motility disturbance. Then it is nearly certain that it is not due to involvement of the third nerve.

* Establish whether segmental palsy of the iris sphincter is present or not. If it is, then the cause is either a postganglionic parasympathetic denervation (eg, acute Adie's pupil—deep tendon reflexes may also be diminished but not always) or less commonly, direct damage to some segments of the iris sphincter from ischemia or trauma.

* When there is no segmental asymmetry of pupil constriction, then suspect either pharmacologic mydriasis (anticholinergic or sympathomimetic) or sympathetic overactivation associated with migraine.

Bibliography

Jacobson DM. Benign episodic unilateral mydriasis: clinical characteristics. *Ophthalmology.* 1995;102(11):1623-1627.

Kardon RH. Disturbances of the pupil. In: Noseworthy JH, ed. *Neurological Therapeutics Principles and Practice.* 2nd ed. Oxon, UK: Informa Healthcare; 2006:1981-1997.

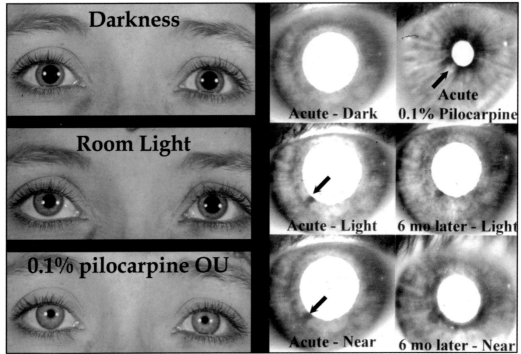

Figure 24-1. Patient with unilateral left mydriasis that is more apparent in light (middle) compared to darkness (top). Addition of dilute 0.1% pilocarpine causes both pupils to constrict, but left pupil constricts more, indicating cholinergic supersensitivity. Infrared transillumination of the iris in the acute state of postganglionic denervation due to Adie's pupil (right panel of monochrome photos, acute). In darkness, the entire sphincter is at rest and has no density except light gray in the pupillary border area. With either light (middle left) or near effort (lower left), only the normal sphincter segment at the 7 o'clock meridian contracts, causing it to appear darker. The other segments are denervated and do not move to light or near and therefore, do not change in density. After dilute 0.1% pilocarpine (top right), all of the nonworking segments that are supersensitive are contracted, even in darkness, causing them to now appear dark. Only the normal segment at the 7 o'clock meridian is not supersensitive and stays light gray in darkness. Aberrant regeneration with light near dissociation has started to take place after 6 months, causing some pupil constriction even in darkness (middle right) and even more contraction with near effort (bottom right).

Kardon RH, Corbett JJ, Thompson HS. Segmental denervation and reinnervation of the iris sphincter as shown by infrared videographic transillumination. *Ophthalmology.* 1998;105:313-321.

Sarkies NJ, Sanders MD, Gautier-Smith PC. Episodic unilateral mydriasis and migraine. *Am J Ophthalmol.* 1985; 99(2):217-218.

Thompson HS, Newsome DA, Loewenfeld IE. The fixed dilated pupil: sudden iridoplegia or mydriatic drops? A simple diagnostic test. *Arch Ophthalmol.* 1971;86:21.

WHAT IS THE EVALUATION FOR
EPISODIC ANISOCORIA?

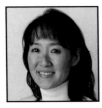

Aki Kawasaki, MD

A 45-year-old-man was noted by his wife to have an extremely large right pupil. He complains of some visual blurring in the right eye but denies any diplopia or toxic exposures. By the time he is evaluated 4 days later, the pupils are now equal in size and reactivity, his vision is normal, and he has normal motility. What are the possible causes for his transient pupil dilation?

When a patient has episodic anisocoria, the initial dilemma lies in deciding which is the abnormal pupil: the larger one or the smaller one? In most cases, we must rely on a descriptive account of accompanying symptoms or signs such as visual blur, pain, ptosis, impaired eye movement, and conjunctival injection to best guess the side of the abnormal pupil. In the patient described above, a history of visual blur in his right eye suggests that his dilated right pupil was indeed the faulty pupil. Because acute mydriasis is a finding that raises the anxiety level of most clinicians, let us first consider some of the oft-invoked neurologic diagnoses in the context of our patient.

Brain herniation? No. It is true that pupillary dilation may herald transtentorial herniation of the brain but in such a setting, the patient is usually comatose with various neurologic deficits. Our patient is awake, alert, and neurologically intact.

Cerebral aneurysm? No. His mydriasis was transient, as confirmed by examination. Episodic dilation of a pupil that recovers completely between episodes is never an aneurysm. Additionally, the patient had no signs of an oculomotor nerve palsy (eg, no ptosis, no ophthalmoplegia). For all practical purposes, an isolated unilateral mydriasis is not due to an aneurysm and is highly unlikely to be the sole manifestation of an oculomotor nerve palsy of any cause.

Seizure? No. Seizure-related mydriasis is associated with an abrupt change in mental status as well as involuntary contraversive head or eye movements. It is an extremely rare occurrence.

Thus, the isolated occurrence and transient duration of a unilateral mydriasis are reassuring features that essentially rule out serious intracranial disease.

What then are possible causes of a transiently dilated pupil?

Intermittent angle-closure glaucoma must be excluded. A history of periorbital pain or headache and blurred vision, particularly seeing halos around lights, accompanying pupillary dilation is highly suggestive. The patient may notice that the affected eye is red and tender to touch during the episode. Gonioscopy is diagnostic.

Paroxysmal discharge of irritated cervical sympathetic nerves is a rare cause of episodic unilateral mydriasis. Other signs of sympathetic hyperactivity, notably lid retraction, conjunctival blanching, and facial hyperhidrosis, are usually present. Visual blur is not a common feature. This phenomenon has been described in occasional patients with disease of the cervical spine, upper cord, brachial plexus, or lung apex. Neck and chest imaging is recommended for patients with symptoms referable to these areas. Some of these patients later develop an ipsilateral oculosympathetic deficit (Horner syndrome), presumably related to progressive damage to the nerves.

Tad-pole–shaped pupil is a related entity. Pupillary distortion with a pointy peak on one side results from focal spasm of the iris dilator muscle. Look for an underlying Horner syndrome.

Pharmacologic mydriasis usually occurs from inadvertent contact with plants containing belladonna alkaloids, such as jimsonweed (thornapple), angel's trumpet, deadly nightshade, and black henbane. These plants may be cultivated in gardens or found growing wild along roadsides and in fields (eg, cornpicker's mydriasis). The degree of pupil dilation and loss of reactivity to light varies depending on the amount of plant alkaloid exposure. A similar degree of accommodative paresis accompanies the mydriasis. Systemic symptoms such as tachycardia, flushing, and dry mouth are rare in cases of local (ocular) exposure. In the acute stage of intoxication, the diagnosis is made from a history of plant contact and the absence of pupillary constriction to topical 1% pilocarpine. In all cases, the mydriasis resolves in 1 to 7 days.

Accidental ocular exposure to bronchodilating mists due to an ill-fitting aerosol mask is an occasional cause of a fixed and dilated pupil in a hospitalized patient. A correct diagnosis in this setting will spare everyone the stress, effort, and cost of an urgent neurologic evaluation.

Migraine can be associated with transient anisocoria but the mechanism is not fully established and is likely multifactorial. In some patients, migrainous vasospasm causing reversible ischemia of the ciliary ganglion leads to a dilated, poorly reactive pupil and accommodative palsy. In others, sympathetic dysregulation, occurring either as increased or decreased activity, has been described. Anisocoria during migraine may also be an exaggerated form of a physiologic anisocoria.

Benign episodic mydriasis is a descriptive term for recurrent episodes of isolated unilateral mydriasis, usually in young women with migraines. The mydriasis typically appears in the same eye but can alternate sides; it may occur during a migraine or independent of headache. The duration of mydriasis is usually several hours but may persist for days. When examined during an episode, some patients have a normal pupil light reflex whereas others show a poor light response with impaired accommodation. Some patients complain of visual blur; others have orbital pain or red eye. Benign episodic mydriasis probably represents a heterogeneous group of disorders, including migraine, having different mechanisms that result in transient unilateral mydriasis. It is called benign because it is not associated with any systemic or neurologic condition.

The patient described in the above case falls under the rubric of benign episodic mydriasis. Given a normal neurologic and ophthalmologic examination, including gonioscopy, no further investigations are currently needed.

Summary

* The isolated occurrence and transient duration of a unilateral mydriasis are reassuring features that essentially rule out serious intracranial disease.

* Benign episodic mydriasis is a descriptive term for recurrent episodes of isolated unilateral mydriasis, usually in young women with migraines. The duration of the mydriasis is usually several hours but it may persist for days.

Bibliography

Jacobson DM. Benign episodic unilateral mydriasis: clinical characteristics. *Ophthalmology*. 1995;102:1623-1627.
Miller NR. Intermittent pupillary dilation in a young woman. *Surv Ophthalmol*. 1986;31:65-68.
Woods D, O'Connor PS, Fleming R. Episodic unilateral mydriasis and migraine. *Am J Ophthalmol*. 1984;98:229-234.

26

HOW DO YOU MANAGE TOXIC AND NUTRITIONAL OPTIC NEUROPATHIES?

Julie Falardeau, MD, FRCSC

A 24-year-old man has been referred for progressive bilateral visual loss. On Thanksgiving of 2002 he noted blurring of vision OU especially affecting central vision. He described a "hole" in his vision bilaterally as if a "light bulb went off" in vision centrally. There has been no exposure to toxins or animals, eye pain, or headaches. He smokes one pack of cigarettes daily (for the past 5 years), drinks 24 beers or more weekly, and lives on his own and does not eat regular meals. There is no family history of ophthalmologic diseases. His exam reveals visual acuity of 20/200 OD and 20/400 OS. There are bilateral cecocentral scotomas and the optic nerves are pale temporally bilaterally. What diagnoses should be considered?

Toxic and nutritional optic neuropathies are typically characterized by bilateral, simultaneous visual impairment with progressive loss of visual acuity, dyschromatopsia, central or cecocentral scotoma, papillomacular bundle damage, and temporal optic disc atrophy. When a patient presents with this constellation of signs, a thorough history is crucial. An extensive history may be the best way to uncover the circumstances that involve toxic/nutritional optic neuropathy. I would emphasize diet, tobacco and alcohol use, and drug and toxin exposure. Treatment of any chronic illness or disease should be elucidated.

Nutritional optic neuropathy typically involves deficiencies in vitamin B_{12} (cobalamin), vitamin B_1 (thiamine), vitamin B_2 (riboflavin), and folic acid. Optic neuropathies from pure nutritional deficiencies have been reported in strict vegan patients. Certain weight reduction methods, including gastric bypass surgery, may result in deficits of

---

Table 26-1
Agents Associated With Toxic Optic Neuropathy

Alpha-interferon 2b	Dapsone	Melatonin
Amiodarone	Digitalis	Methanol
Carbon monoxide	Disulfiram	Perchloroethylene
Carboplatin	Ethambutol	Quinine
Chloramphenicol	Ethylene glycol	Sertraline
Chloroquine	5-Fluorouracil	Streptomycin
Cimetidine	Isoniazid	Sulfonamides
Cisplatin	Lead	Tacrolimus
Cyclosporine	Linezolid	Toluene
		Vincristine

---

vitamins and can be complicated by vision loss from bilateral optic neuropathy. Vitamin B$_{12}$ deficiency is the most common cause of nutritional amblyopia and generally arises in 3 different clinical settings: 1) pernicious anemia, 2) previous history of partial or complete stomach or ileum removal, and 3) strict vegan diet. Since optic neuropathies due solely to nutritional deficiencies remain rare in North America, it is important to ask about tobacco use and alcohol consumption. Nutritional optic neuropathy is clearly more common among tobacco and alcohol abusers. Numerous other agents have also been identified as a potential cause of toxic optic neuropathy through presumed direct metabolic impairments but the main one to consider is ethambutol (Table 26-1).

Progressive dimness of vision is the classic symptom. Patients become aware of gradual blurred central vision that is slowly progressive. This visual loss is painless, bilateral, and simultaneous though the involvement can be asymmetric in the acute phase. Color vision should be tested since dyschromatopsia is a constant feature and occurs early. There is usually no relative afferent pupillary defect since the disease is almost always bilateral and symmetric. Most patients will present with normal-appearing optic discs in the early stages. Optic disc edema may be seen in some toxic optic neuropathies such as those caused by amiodarone and isoniazid toxicity. Papillomacular bundle loss and optic atrophy (especially temporal atrophy) finally develop in the chronic stages. Formal visual field testing with either static or kinetic perimetry is essential in the evaluation of a patient suspected of suffering from toxic/nutritional optic neuropathy. Bilateral central or cecocentral scotomas with preservation of the peripheral visual field are characteristic of these optic neuropathies.

A family history of bilateral vision loss should be noted and investigated since Leber's hereditary optic neuropathy can present in a similar way. A detailed review of the system should inquire about peripheral sensory symptoms and gait disturbance because these might reflect a nutritional/toxic peripheral neuropathy.

The differential diagnosis of toxic/nutritional optic neuropathy may be challenging. Other conditions should be considered, including the following:

* Compressive optic neuropathy
* Leber's hereditary optic neuropathy
* Dominant inherited optic neuropathy
* Maculopathy/macular dystrophy
* Syphilitic optic neuropathy
* Radiation optic neuropathy
* Bilateral inflammatory or demyelinating optic neuropathy
* Infiltrative optic neuropathy

I would suggest that your patient undergo laboratory studies, including a complete blood count with differential, serum B_{12}, red blood cell folate, and syphilis serology. Leber's mitochondrial DNA mutation testing and heavy metal screening should be considered if the etiology remains unknown after the initial work-up. Since there are many examples of bilateral cecocentral scotoma secondary to compressive or infiltrative lesions, a neuroimaging study should be performed even if toxic/nutritional optic neuropathy is highly suspected. Magnetic resonance imaging (MRI) with and without contrast enhancement and fat suppression remains the study of choice to rule out a compressive or infiltrative process involving the optic chiasm or optic nerves.

The first step in managing toxic optic neuropathy is to remove the offending agent. This may cause some reversal of the process, especially if removed early in the course of the optic nerve dysfunction. Other than stopping the drug, no specific treatment is available for these optic neuropathies. For patients in whom the diagnosis of tobacco-alcohol amblyopia is suspected, it cannot be overemphasized that stopping, or at least reducing, tobacco and alcohol consumption is critical to their recovery. For nutritional optic neuropathies, improved nutrition is essential. I strongly recommend comanaging these patients with an internist. Medical therapy includes vitamin supplementation with thiamine, folic acid, multivitamins, and, in case of pernicious anemia, vitamin B_{12} injections monthly for several months. The elimination of any causative agent such as alcohol is also a key factor for potential recovery. The visual prognosis is typically poor if optic atrophy is already present.

I think that most likely your patient has a nutritional optic neuropathy and needs to quit smoking and stop alcohol consumption. In a young man with this clinical picture, however, Leber's hereditary optic neuropathy is also of concern.

Summary

* Toxic and nutritional optic neuropathies are typically characterized by bilateral, simultaneous visual impairment with progressive loss of visual acuity, dyschromatopsia, central or cecocentral scotoma, papillomacular bundle damage, and temporal optic disc atrophy.

* Since bilateral cecocentral scotoma may occur secondary to compressive or infiltrative lesions, a neuroimaging study should be performed even if toxic/nutritional optic neuropathy is highly suspected.

* Leber's mitochondrial DNA mutation testing should be considered if the etiology of a presumed toxic/nutritional optic neuropathy remains unknown after the initial work-up.

Bibliography

Lloyd MJ, Fraunfelder FW. Drug-induced optic neuropathies. *Drugs Today.* 2007;43:829-838.

Orsaaud C, Roche O, Dufier JL. Nutritional optic neuropathies. *J Neurol Sci.* 2007;262:158-164.

Phillips PH. Toxic and deficiency optic neuropathies. In: Miller NR, Newman NJ, eds. *Walsh and Hoyt's Clinical Neuro-Ophthalmology.* 6th ed. Baltimore, MD: Lippincott Williams & Wilkins; 2005:447-463.

Sadun AA. Metabolic optic neuropathies. *Semin Ophthalmol.* 2002;17:29-32.

27

WHAT ARE VISUAL PROCESSING DEFECTS AND HOW CAN I RECOGNIZE THEM?

Swaraj Bose, MD

A 70-year-old man who complains of a 5-year history of visual difficulty is being examined. He has been having trouble driving and has gotten in many accidents, although eye exams have been said to be "normal." Recently he fell off of a fishing pier because he "did not notice the ocean." He also noted difficulty in cutting his food and in reaching for objects. On ophthalmologic examination his vision was intact with no significant visual field impairment. He missed all of the H-R-R color plates bilaterally, although he was able to name all of the colors on the plates correctly. He had difficulty in describing the complete contents of a picture although he could describe parts of the picture accurately. He had retained insight, a good sense of humor, and a relatively intact mental status otherwise. What is likely causing his visual impairment?

My first reaction listening to the case would be does this gentleman suffer from an organic or a nonorganic (functional) vision loss? The next step should be to determine the possible anatomical location of vision loss: 1) Is it optical in nature? Is something wrong with the focusing elements, like the cornea, lens, or media transparency?, 2) Is there a problem with the retinocortical component? This includes problems in the retina, optic nerve, chiasm, optic tract, lateral geniculate body, optic radiations, and the primary visual cortex, or 3) Is this a problem with the visual integration or processing mechanism? These include occipito-parietal or occipito-temporal pathway lesions or problems with visual attention and object recognition. There are clues in the history that suggest he is suffering from an organic cause rather than demonstrating a case of functional visual loss. Our patient has a history of repeated accidents, normal eye examination including visual acuity and fields, normal mental status, with a reduced response to stimuli presented either side of fixation (difficulty in cutting food, reaching for objects, missing color plates) and a reduced ability to detect one visual object at the same time, and an inability to combine several viewed objects into a meaningful composite (difficulty in describing the complete contents of the picture but describes parts of the picture accurately). A combination of these findings suggests that there is a problem with visual integration and processing as the cause of his visual disturbances. The diagnosis is bilateral visual inattention or "simultagnosia."

Such patients with simultagnosia complain of piecemeal perception of the visual environment wherein objects may look fragmented or even appear to vanish from direct view. Simultagnosia is caused by a defect in visual attention that results in an inability to sustain visuospatial processing across simultaneous elements in an array. This is a higher disorder of visual processing and attention and may result from bilateral superior parieto-occipital lobe strokes, occlusion of posterior cerebral arteries usually occurring after systemic hypotensive crises, cardiac arrest, Alzheimer's disease (visual variant), and intraoperative hypotension. A similar case has also been described following lumboperitoneal shunt for pseudotumor cerebri. Experimental and clinical studies have confirmed that the parieto-occipital areas are activated during visual attentional tasks. Simultagnosia occurs in 2 distinct settings: 1) hypoxic and hypotensive injuries in the distribution of the posterior cerebral circulation and 2) Alzheimer's disease. In contrast to the typical case of Alzheimer's disease, a visual variant has been described where patients present with predominantly visual symptoms including homonymous visual field defects resulting from involvement of the visual association cortex. These patients have a normal eye exam but demonstrate atrophy of the parieto-occipital regions in magnetic resonance imaging (MRI) scans while those with a normal brain MRI show hypoperfusion in the parieto-occipital regions in functional neuroimaging (positron emission tomography [PET] scans, functional MRI [fMRI]).

The presenting complaints usually include tunnel vision, bumping into objects, trouble reading and interpreting pictures, loss of depth perception, and objects fading in and out of sight. Eye examination including visual acuity, pupils, anterior segment examination, and fundus are normal. Visual fields are quite constricted. Visual stimuli may suddenly appear and disappear from fixation even as the eyes continue to stare at the stimulus. Like in our patient, observing the patient while performing an Ishihara or H-R-R color test is a good and reliable test for simultagnosia where the patient usually misses all color plates but is able to name the colors perfectly well. Another clue to diagnosis is the large discrepancy between relatively intact fields to cued, single-finger confrontation without an interesting fixation target and depressed visual fields to uncued, standard multiple-finger confrontation or automated field testing. Also, these patients typically do not have problems reading individual letters, while they make numerous errors with words and sentences. Interpreting detailed pictures is also an issue; they can identify individual components but cannot identify their interactions. For example, in a patient when handed a dollar bill, he identified George Washington but could not identify the money! Other simple diagnostic tests include difficulty in counting arrays of objects without proprioceptive input from their fingers, they walk very cautiously and walk into large and previously viewed objects, and they cannot move their eyes to targets in extrapersonal visual space.

Table 27-1

Screening Tests for Patients With Visual Processing Defects

Navigation	Patients with bilateral visual inattention walk hesitatingly in short, slow steps, with outstretched arms (like a blind person) and collide with objects previously noted to be there. Can be difficult to distinguish from the one with functional visual loss. Other tests should be used in conjunction.
Confrontation visual fields	Initially present single fingers and the patient is able to identify single fingers then present 2 fingers in the same quadrant, and a persistence of failure to notice both fingers suggests visual inattention in the given quadrant.
Eliminating fixation target	While performing the confrontation visual field, instead of having the patient fixate on your eye, have him gaze ahead on a space (eg, the wall), repeat the test as above (#2). The peripheral stimuli will be more easily identified when there is no competing fixation target, suggesting visual inattention.
Color plate tests	Using the Ishihara or H-R-R plates, the patient is usually unable to identify the numbers; however, he or she is able to recognize the individual colors.
Counting arrays	After the patient correctly identifies an object like a pen, show him or her 4 or 5 pens in an array and instruct him or her to count by sight. If unsuccessful, ask him or her to touch and count the pens; if this tactile contact improves the counting accuracy, visual inattention is a possibility.
Reading	Errors in reading like compressing, omitting single words or parts, or jumbling the order of words suggest visual and spatial inattention.
Interpreting pictures	A failure to interpret the scene while correctly identifying the individual components in a magazine picture denotes visual inattention.

Patients suffering from visual attention syndromes and simultagnosia are usually misdiagnosed as functional visual loss and see a number of physicians before a diagnosis is established. Early recognition and a referral to a neuro-ophthalmologist is a key to early management. The treating physician should obtain an excellent history, demonstrate a negative anterior and posterior segment eye examination, and perform screening tests including visual field testing (Table 27-1). Other tests like neuropsychological testing (if you suspect Alzheimer's disease), neuroimaging including a brain MRI and magnetic resonance angiography (MRA) and possibly functional neuroimaging (including PET and fMRI) in cases with negative MRI scans may be needed to establish an accurate diagnosis. I would like to emphasize that all patients do not need functional neuroimaging to establish a diagnosis and we should keep cost effectiveness in mind. Treatment strategies should be directed toward etiology and neurorehabilitation.

Summary

* Patients with lesions of the parietal vision-related cortex present with deficits related to the distribution of visual attention and the perception and manipulation of items in space.

* Those with unilateral lesions usually confine their attention to the ipsilateral hemisphere and those with bilateral occipito-parietal lesions keep their eyes fixed on a target, walk cautiously with outstretched arms, collide with previously seen objects, and behave as if they have searchlight vision.

* These patients should be distinguished from nonorganic or functional blindness and although they are usually not considered blind based on standard vision tests, functionally they are severely visually impaired.

Bibliography

Lee AG, Martin CO. Neuro-ophthalmic findings in the visual variant of Alzheimer's disease. *Ophthalmology.* 2004; 111:376-381.

Miller NR. Bilateral visual loss and simultagnosia after lumboperitoneal shunt for pseudotumor cerebri. *J Neuroophthalmol.* 1997;17:36-38.

Poggel DA, Kasten E, Muller-Oehring EM, Bunzenthal U, Sabel BA. Improving residual vision by attentional cueing in patients with brain lesions. *Brain Res.* 2006;1097:142-148.

Trobe JR, ed. *The Neurology of Vision.* New York, NY: Oxford University Press; 2001:334-336.

Wurtz RH, Goldberg ME, Robinson DL. Brain mechanisms of visual attention. *Sci Am.* 1982;246:1-135.

28

How Do I Manage Headache Syndromes That Come to Me as an Ophthalmologist?

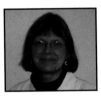

Kathleen B. Digre, MD

A 37-year-old woman who has developed recurrent left-side headaches over the past 2 months is being examined. The pains are located in the left orbital-temporal region, are excruciatingly severe, last 4 to 10 minutes, occur 8 to 15 times per day, and are associated with bilateral conjunctival injection and lacrimation. The neuro-ophthalmologic exam was normal. What entities should be considered as a cause of these paroxysms? What treatments should be considered?

The patient who complains about headache to an ophthalmologist usually wonders if the pain has to do with the eye. A long-lasting (hours-days) unilateral headache that is moderate to severe and associated with nausea and/or vomiting as well as photophobia is usually migraine. However, a short-lasting headache in and around the eye or head with autonomic symptoms can be a vexing problem for any ophthalmologist. The good news is that short-lasting headaches can be diagnosed and treated.

The first problem is recognition that stabbing pains are a "primary headache disorder" and not due to a secondary process. The patient understandably believes that the severe pain occurring in the orbital temporal region is due to a serious problem like a tumor or an aneurysm. Headaches that are due to an underlying process by definition must be excluded. I use the following "rules of thumb" to help me diagnose a secondary headache:

* A new headache in someone who is not otherwise headache prone

* A headache in an older person—always rule out giant cell arteritis

* A side-locked headache that never goes away—needs imaging

* A headache associated with neurological findings: Horner syndrome (rule out carotid dissection), weakness, numbness, diplopia
* A headache that awakens someone in the middle of the night provided it is not a cluster or other trigeminal autonomic cephalgia
* Eye diseases that could present with episodic eye pain include glaucoma and trochleitis (usually find tenderness over the trochlea). Other eye disorders like early Zoster ophthalmicus, optic neuritis, and posterior scleritis will not have episodic eye pain but may have pain as the presenting symptom

In many of the stabbing headache syndromes, imaging studies may have been performed before you see the patient. If not, or you are in doubt, consider ordering magnetic resonance imaging (MRI) for these short stabbing headaches to be sure there is no abnormality in the pituitary gland, cavernous sinus, or skull base.

Fortunately, most recurrent stabbing or throbbing pains are primary headache disorders. The next job is to diagnose the headache type. The clues to look for are symptoms of autonomic dysfunction: ptosis, eyelid edema, lacrimation, rhinorrhea, red eye, possibly an intermittent Horner syndrome (with ptosis, miosis), and conjunctival injection. If the patient has any one of these symptoms along with episodic unilateral pain in and around the eye, chances are the patient has a primary short-lasting headache or "trigeminal autonomic cephalgia." The patient above has conjunctival injection and lacrimation.

Next determine which type of trigeminal autonomic cephalgia the patient has. These headaches divide themselves between the length of the headache, the number of headaches each day, and the gender of the person. In general, cluster headache and short unilateral neuralgiform pain with conjunctival injection and tearing (SUNCT) are more common in men, whereas paroxysmal hemicrania and hemicrania continua are more common in women.

The length of time of the pain is helpful. The longest trigeminal autonomic cephalgia is hemicrania continua. It is characterized by chronic pain on one side of the head with paroxysms of stabbing pain on top of that. The pain can last hours or days. The next longest is cluster headache lasting 20 to 120 minutes. Paroxysmal hemicrania is much shorter, usually 2 to 45 minutes at a time. Short unilateral neuralgiform pain with (SUNCT) or without (SUNA) conjunctival injection and tearing are 15 to 120 seconds each.

Hemicrania continua is by definition continuous. Cluster occurs anywhere between 1 to 3 times each day; most of the time, one of the pains will occur in sleep. Paroxysmal hemicrania occurs usually more than 5 times each day. SUNCT/SUNA can occur 30 times an hour.

Using Table 28-1, we have a woman with 8 to 15 attacks a day lasting 4 to 10 minutes each; this fits with paroxysmal hemicrania.

Preventative treatment with indomethacin is always worth a try in many of these short-lasting headaches. Hemicrania continua and paroxysmal hemicrania have the absolute response to this medication as part of the definition of the headache. Doses of 25 mg 3 times each day to 75 mg slow release form twice each day usually suffice. When indomethacin is not tolerated or can not be used, Cox-2 inhibitors, verapamil, aspirin, and anticonvulsants (gabapentin, topiramate, valproate, lamotrigine) may be used.

Acute treatment of the pain is difficult. Most of the time the headache is so brief that acute treatments will not be helpful. Oxygen can be administered at the onset of the heache (cluster headache usually responds to oxgyen 5-10 L/minute for 10 min) may be

Table 28-1
Distinguishing Trigeminal Autonomic Cephalgias

Headache Type	Gender	Length of Headache	Frequency	Response to Indomethacin
Hemicrania continua	Female>male	Continuous	Multiple stabbing pains on top of continuous headache	Complete
Paroxysmal hemicrania	Female>male	4 to 15 minutes	>5 day; nocturnal headache	Complete
Cluster headache	Male>female	30 to 120 minutes	1 to 5/day; often nocturnal onset	Rarely helpful
SUNCT	Male>female	5 to 250 seconds	1/day to 30/hour	Rarely helpful
SUNA	Male>female	5 to 250 seconds	1/day to 30/hour	Rarely helpful

helpful. Also in cluster headache because it lasts longer, trials of intranasal triptans such as sumatriptan, zolmitriptan, or injectable sumatriptan may be useful.

Your patient probably has paroxysmal hemicrania. She probably will need to be referred to a neurologist to try specific medication treatments for this entity.

Summary

* Although most recurrent stabbing or throbbing headaches are primary headache disorders, always consider secondary headache or eye pain symdromes.

* In many of the stabbing headache syndromes, imaging studies may have been performed before you see the patient. If not, or you are in doubt, order an MRI for these short stabbing headaches to be sure there is no abnormality in the pituitary gland, cavernous sinus, or skull base.

* It is important to look for symptoms of autonomic dysfunction in patients with unilateral headache or eye pain. These symptoms include ptosis, eyelid edema, lacrimation, rhinorrhea, red eye, possibly an intermittent Horner's syndrome (with ptosis, miosis), and conjunctival injection. If the patient has any one of these symptoms along with episodic unilateral pain in and around the eye, chances are the patient has a primary short-lasting headache or trigeminal autonomic cephalgia.

* Trigeminal autonomic cephalgias are defined by the length of the headache, the number of headaches each day, and the gender of the person.

Bibliography

Cohen AS, Matharu MS, Goadsby PJ. Trigeminal autonomic cephalgias: current and future treatments. *Headache.* 2007;47:969-980.

Favier I, van Vliet JA, Roon KI, et al. Trigeminal autonomic cephalgias due to structural lesions: a review of 31 cases. *Arch Neurol.* 2007;64:25-31.

Friedman DI. The eye and headache. *Ophthalmol Clin North Am.* 2004;17:357-369.

May A. Update on the diagnosis and management of trigemino-autonomic headaches. *J Neurol.* 2006;253:1525-1532.

WHAT IS THE EVALUATION OF OPTIC ATROPHY?

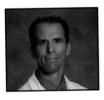

Karl C. Golnik, MD, MEd

A 47-year-old patient with impaired vision and optic atrophy bilaterally was seen for routine eye examination. What etiologies should be considered? What is the likelihood of discovering a treatable etiology for the atrophy?

Optic disc pallor and *atrophy* are terms used synonymously, but there is a wide range of "normal" color of the disc. If true atrophy (damage) exists, it should be accompanied by visual loss (acuity and/or peripheral vision), decreased color perception (if acuity is compromised), and a relative afferent pupillary defect if the atrophy is unilateral. I will assume that your patient has no other cause of visual loss and that true optic atrophy exists. Primary optic nerve damage is our first consideration, but you should keep in mind that retinal damage (eg, old vascular event, retinitis pigmentosa) can also result in optic atrophy.

A complete ophthalmic examination including a comprehensive history will lead to an underlying diagnosis in the vast majority of optic atrophy cases. The most common etiologies of optic neuropathy, non-arteritic anterior ischemic optic neuropathy (NAION) and optic neuritis, are also the most common causes of optic atrophy. Your patient is 47 years old, a "gray zone" for differential diagnosis by age, and thus either previous ischemia or inflammation is possible. If there was sudden, painless visual loss, I would lean toward a vascular etiology; if it was subacute painful visual loss, then perhaps inflammation had occurred whereas gradual visual loss may indicate a compressive or nutritional etiology. One caveat, however, is that sudden discovery of chronic monocular visual loss may confound the history. Optic atrophy develops several months after damage and thus

Figure 29-1. Note the superior altitudinal optic atrophy in a patient with previous NAION.

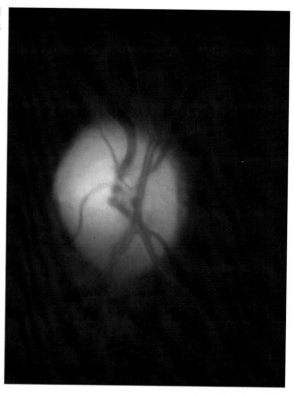

the patient who presents with acute or subacute visual loss (days to several weeks) and optic atrophy must have a more chronic process. If there has been no change in vision since the loss, then I would favor previous ischemia or trauma whereas progressive visual loss may indicate continued damage from compression or nutritional deficits. Old records documenting prior disc swelling would indicate probable prior NAION.

Past medical illnesses, such as multiple sclerosis, severe vascular disease, sarcoidosis, or malignancy, may suggest the cause of the optic atrophy. History of focal paresthesias or weakness may indicate demyelinating disease and shortness of breath and/or skin rash may occur with sarcoidosis. Gradual bilateral visual loss in other family members suggests possible dominant optic atrophy whereas a maternal family history suggests Leber's hereditary optic neuropathy. Finally, toxic exposures (methanol), contact with animals (cats, ticks), medications (ethambutol), and vitamin deficiencies (history of alcoholism) may direct diagnostic evaluation.

You should look carefully for clues in the ophthalmologic exam that may aid in determining the underlying etiology of optic atrophy. Anterior segment exam may reveal evidence of previous trauma such as iris tears. Additionally, the presence of active or previous inflammation such as keratic precipitates or vitreous cell may point toward an infectious or inflammatory cause of optic atrophy such as sarcoid, syphilis, cat-scratch disease, or Lyme disease. Formal visual field testing may detect specific patterns of visual loss helpful in the differential diagnosis. Central scotomas occur more commonly in nutritional, hereditary, or toxic optic neuropathies. Hemianopic field deficits suggest chiasmal or retrochiasmal damage.

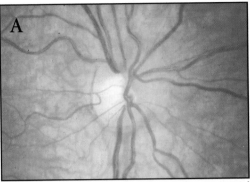
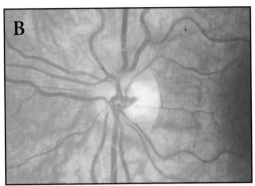

Figure 29-2. Note the band atrophy present in the left disc and temporal atrophy in the right disc of a patient with a right optic tract glioma.

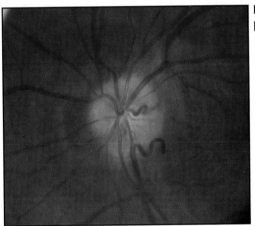

Figure 29-3. Optociliary collateral vessels in a patient with an optic nerve sheath meningioma.

Although diffuse optic atrophy is nonspecific, examination may reveal subtle clues about causes of the optic atrophy. An altitudinally atrophic disc is most often seen in NAION (Figure 29-1). Remember to confirm that the contralateral disc is small and congested (the disc-at-risk) when entertaining the diagnosis of NAION. Horizontal band (or "bow-tie") atrophy may be present with optic chiasmal or retrochiasmal pregeniculate lesions (Figure 29-2). Optociliary collateral vessels may become apparent when retinal venous outflow is compromised by an optic nerve sheath meningioma (Figure 29-3). Of course, one must examine the nerve with slit lamp biomicroscopy to obtain a good three-dimensional view and to rule out subtle cupping that might occur in glaucoma.

Laboratory testing such as angiotension-converting enzyme, FTA-ABS, Lyme titer, and cat-scratch titer (Bartonella henselae), Leber's hereditary optic neuropathy, or dominant optic atrophy (OPA1) may prove useful but only when history or examination (as described above) has suggested the possibility of one of these diseases. I do not recommend "shot-gun" testing for isolated optic atrophy without cause from history or exam. Lab tests for infectious causes of optic atrophy can produce false-positive results and are not useful without clinical correlation.

Recently, we reported imaging results of a series of patients referred with unexplained, isolated, unilateral optic atrophy. Twenty percent of these patients had compressive lesions demonstrated by magnetic resonance imaging (MRI) with fat suppression and gadolinium administration. Thus, if our patient has no clues in the history or examination and has seen his or her family physician for physical examination, I would obtain MRI with gadolinium and fat suppression. If an MRI has been previously obtained, then I would review the films.

Unfortunately, I do not always discover a definite cause of the atrophy. If our patient's evaluation conducted as described above is negative, then I would recommend repeating the evaluation with automated perimetry in 3 months to be sure there is no progressive loss of vision. If the exam is stable, I would see the patient on several occasions over the next 2 years to prove stability. If vision worsened during follow-up, I would consider progressive entities such as compression, nutritional deficiency, and dominant optic atrophy and investigate further.

Summary

* Examination including a comprehensive history will lead to an underlying diagnosis in approximately 92% of cases of optic atrophy.

* Optic atrophy develops several months after damage and thus the patient who presents with acute or subacute visual loss (days to several weeks) and optic atrophy must have a more chronic process.

* The most common etiologies of optic neuropathy, NAION and optic neuritis, are also the most common causes of optic atrophy.

* In a neuroimaging study of 91 patients referred with unexplained, isolated, unilateral optic atrophy, 20% of patients had compressive lesions demonstrated by MRI with fat suppression and gadolinium administration.

Bibliography

Bakken L, Callister S, Wand P. Interlaboratory comparison of test results for detection of Lyme disease in 516 participants in the Wisconsin State Laboratory of Hygiene/College of American Pathologists Proficiency Testing Program. *J Clin Microbiol.* 1997;35:537-543.

Lee A, Chau F, Golnik K, Kardon R, Wall M. The diagnostic yield of the evaluation for isolated unexplained optic atrophy. *Ophthalmology.* 2005;112:757-759.

Sander A, Posselt M, Oberle K. Seroprevalence of antibodies to Bartonellae henselae in patients with cat-scratch disease and in healthy controls: evaluation and comparison of two commercial serological tests. *Clinical and Diagnostic Laboratory Immunology.* 1998;5:486-490.

WHAT DO I DO IN A CHILD WITH ASYMMETRIC NYSTAGMUS?

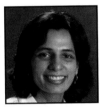

Madhura A. Tamhankar, MD
(co-authored with Grant T. Liu, MD)

A 2-year-old child who was noted by his mother to have "jumping" eyes is being examined. On exam there is a pendular intermittent unilateral nystagmus of high frequency and small amplitude with a "shimmering" quality. The nystagmus is mainly horizontal with a torsional component. It is associated with irregular head nodding and the patient often also demonstrates a head tilt. What is the likely cause of the abnormalities? Should neuroimaging be performed?

The clinical scenario described in this 2-year-old child is that of a spasmus nutans-like condition. True spasmus nutans is a benign nystagmus that is composed of a triad of nystagmus, head nodding, and torticollis. It begins in the first year of life, usually after 6 months, and spontaneously remits in 1 to 2 years. It consists of pendular oscillations of low amplitude and high frequency (above 7 Hz) that may be unilateral or bilateral but asymmetric. It is usually intermittent and is described as shimmering. It is mostly a horizontal nystagmus but vertical and rotary components can be present. True isolated and idiopathic spasmus nutans is not accompanied by any neurologic abnormalities although strabismus and amblyopia may coexist.

The diagnosis of spasmus nutans is one of exclusion. Groups of spasmus nutans-like conditions exist that mimic the clinically observed signs of spasmus nutans and yet are secondary to sensory defects, either intracranial tumors or retinal degenerative conditions. A number of reports in the literature have documented a spasmus nutans-like nystagmus with hypothalamic and parasellar tumors such as optic pathway glioma. Other signs of afferent visual pathway dysfunction such as visual acuity loss, visual field defects, optic disc atrophy, endocrinologic disturbances, and signs and symptoms of raised intracranial pressure may be present in these patients. One large retrospective series of 67 children presenting with spasmus nutans found no child with intracranial abnormalities although not all the children obtained neuroimaging. Given the reported literature on the presence of hypothalamic and chiasmal gliomas in children presenting with spasmus nutans-like nystagmus, we would obtain magnetic resonance imaging (MRI) of the brain in this or any other patient presenting with spasmus nutans-like nystagmus to exclude intracranial structural abnormalities.

Spasmus nutans-like nystagmus and head movements have also been described in association with retinal diseases such as congenital stationary night blindness and in spinocerebellar degenerations. Some authors have suggested that children presenting with spasmus nutans-like conditions should have an electroretinogram routinely to rule out sensory causes for the nystagmus. Smith et al found abnormal electroretinogram in 3 out of 8 children who presented with spasmus nutans-like nystagmus that was consistent with cone-rod dystrophy in 2 and rod dystrophy in one patient. We currently perform an electroretinogram in patients presenting with asymmetric acquired nystagmus only if the clinical suspicion for retinal dystrophy exists such as with subnormal visual acuity and abnormal ophthalmic examination as detailed above.

It is important to know that although true spasmus nutans is thought to be self-limited, the visual outcome of patients with spasmus nutans is unclear. Although good visual acuity can be expected in patients with spasmus nutans, abnormal stereo acuity, latent nystagmus, strabismus, and amblyopia may develop in the long term.

Summary

* Horizontal asymmetric nystagmus usually occurs in 1 of 3 situations: 1) secondary to an intracranial lesion, 2) with monocular visual loss, or 3) as part of the triad that constitutes the diagnosis of spasmus nutans (asymmetric nystagmus, abnormal head posture, head shake).

* In addition to detailed history taking and clinical examination for systemic abnormalities, neuroimaging is suggested in all children presenting with this type of nystagmus to exclude intracranial space-occupying lesions.

* Electroretinography is reserved for those children in whom clinical suspicion for a retinal dystrophy exists based on history and ophthalmic examination.

Bibliography

Arnoldi KA, Tychsen L. Prevalence of intracranial lesions in children initially diagnosed with disconjugate nystagmus (spasmus nutans). *J Pediatr Ophthalmol Strabismus*. 1995;32:296-301. Erratum in: *J Pediatr Ophthalmol Strabismus*. 1995;32:347.

Farmer J, Hoyt CS. Monocular nystagmus in infancy and early childhood. *Am J Ophthalmol*. 1984;98:504-509.

Gottlob I, Wizov SS, Reinecke RD. Spasmus nutans: a long-term follow-up. *Invest Ophthalmol Vis Sci*. 1995;36: 2768-2771.

Lavery MA, O'Neill JF, Chu FC, Martyn LJ. Acquired nystagmus in early childhood: a presenting sign of intracranial tumor. *Ophthalmology*. 1984;91:425-453.

Smith DE, Fitzgerald K, Stass-Isern M, Cibis GW. Electroretinography is necessary for spasmus nutans diagnosis. *Pediatr Neurol*. 2000;23:33-36.

WHAT IS OPSOCLONUS AND HOW DO I MANAGE IT?

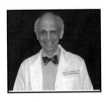

Steve Newman, MD

A 56-year-old man complains that his eyes are "jumping." On exam he has frequent, conjugate, involuntary, large amplitude saccades in all directions. What is the likely cause and what evaluation is warranted?

It is likely that this patient also complains of oscillopsia. This perception of the world jumping is often the initiating complaint in patients who are found to have the condition described here. Opsoclonus, also known as "saccadomania," is basically due to a free run of the saccadic burst cell generator, producing conjugate eye movements in all directions. Characteristic of these conjugate eye movements is the lack of normal intersaccadic latency, which usually measures between 200 and 250 milliseconds. Opsoclonus is distinguished from ocular flutter in that opsoclonus may be in all directions while ocular flutter is only horizontal. Both are due to the same mechanism, which is an abnormality in the pause cells that are located within the nucleus raphe interpositus, which normally dampens the free-running burst cells located in the parapontine reticular formation (PPRF).

Opsoclonus usually occurs in 3 settings. In children, approximately 50% are due to the presence of a neuroblastoma. The most common etiology in young adults is demyelinating disease. In older patients, it is most commonly due to paraneoplastic syndromes. Less commonly vertebrobasilar insufficiency with or without brainstem infarcts or mass lesions may produce opsoclonus. The most likely etiology in the 56-year-old gentleman would be paraneoplastic although we cannot exclude the possibility of other brainstem pathology. The key here would be obtaining a history of previous cancer, particularly small cell lung carcinoma, breast carcinoma (somewhat unlikely in a 56-year-old man), or other malignancies. Auto-antibodies may be positive, including anti-Ri, usually associated with cancer of the breast or pelvic organs and less commonly in small cell lung cancer or bladder cancer. Anti-Hu has also been reported, although this would be less common. Anti-Yo and other anti-Purkinje cell antibodies may be found in women with paraneoplastic opsoclonus and cerebellar degeneration associated with cancer of the breast or gynecological organs. Magnetic resonance imaging (MRI) may be appropriate, and a lumbar puncture (LP) may be done to exclude the possibility of an inflammatory or infectious etiology such as viral encephalitis. Rare cases of oscillopsia have been associated with trauma, usually after hypoxia, although the history here would be diagnostic. Toxic causes of opsoclonus have also been reported (eg, due to amitriptyline, lithium, Dilantin [Parke-Davis, Detroit, MI], or cocaine).

If a tumor is identified, treatment of the tumor itself sometimes results in improvement. Unfortunately, opsoclonus often fails to resolve after resecting the neoplasm. Other treatments have included the use of adrenocorticotropin hormone (ACTH), systemic corticosteroids, and clonazepam, which may improve symptoms even if they do not abolish the eye movements. Plasmapheresis does not appear to be effective. Although intravenous immunoglobulin (IVIG) has been tried, it is unclear exactly how much benefit might be expected. Spontaneous improvement in oscillopsia has also been reported.

Summary

* Opsoclonus, also known as "saccadomania," is basically due to a free run of the saccadic burst cell generator, producing conjugate eye movements in all directions.

* Opsoclonus usually occurs in 3 settings: 1) in children, approximately 50% are due to the presence of a neuroblastoma; 2) in young adults, the most common etiology is demyelinating disease; and 3) in older patients, it is most commonly due to paraneoplastic syndromes.

References

Bataller L, Graus F, Saiz A, Vilchez J. Clinical outcome in adult onset idiopathic or paraneoplastic opsoclonus-myoclonus. *Brain*. 2001;124:437-443.

Digre KB. Opsoclonus in adults: report of three cases and a review of the literature. *Arch Ophthalmol*. 1986;43:1165-1175.

Dropcho J, Kline LB, Riser J. Antineuronal (anti-Ri) antibodies in a patient with steroid-responsive opsoclonus-myoclonus. *Neurology*. 1993;43:207-211.

Pranzatelli MR. The neurobiology of the opsoclonus-myoclonus syndrome clinical. *Clin Neuropharmacology*. 1992;15:186-228.

Shams'ili S, Grefkens J, de Leeuw B, et al. Paraneoplastic cerebellar degeneration associated with antineuronal antibodies: analysis of 50 patients. *Brain*. 2003;126:1409-1418.

32

WHAT IS WERNICKE'S ENCEPHALOPATHY AND HOW DOES IT AFFECT THE EYE?

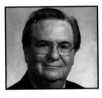

James J. Corbett, MD

A 40-year-old man was seen in the emergency room and was noted to have slowly progressive confusion and imbalance for several days. He is disoriented and confused with an unsteady gait. He has a full range of eye motion and no ocular misalignment. However, he has primary position upbeat nystagmus that becomes downbeat nystagmus with convergence, and mild horizontal end gaze nystagmus. What is the likely etiology of his confusion and eye findings?

In this patient, my major concern would be Wernicke's encephalopathy (WE). This is an organic global confusional ataxic condition usually thought of as seen in alcoholics and caused by thiamine deficiency. Stupor and coma are rarely seen in the initial phase of WE, but untreated WE will progress to stupor, coma, and death in a matter of days. The classic clinical triad of WE includes ataxia, confusion, and ophthalmoplegia. A newer operational definition of the syndrome emphasizes nutritional deficiency as the primary feature. Despite the importance placed on the ocular motor findings in both the classic and revised criteria for diagnosis, the incidence of these clinical findings is relatively low, occurring in only about a quarter to a third of patients studied at necropsy.

The visual problems seen with WE include bilateral, frequently asymmetric ocular motility disturbances and rarely acute nutritional optic neuropathy (Table 32-1). Third and fourth nerve palsies are not reported. Asymmetry of pupil size and impaired light response have also been reported in 19% of patients with WE, but this is the same incidence as simple anisocoria, which occurs in 19% of the population at any given time.

Although classically described in malnourished alcoholics, other conditions are now being cited in association with WE (Table 32-2).

Table 32-1
Ophthalmologic Involvement With Wernicke's Encephalopathy

1. *Horizontal disturbances*

   - Gaze palsy
   - Abduction paresis
   - Vestibular paresis
   - Internuclear ophthalmoplegia
   - Horizontal nystagmus

2. *Vertical disturbances*

   - Upbeat nystagmus (gaze evoked)
   - Downbeat nystagmus (gaze evoked)
   - Skew deviation
   - Mild ptosis (rare)

3. *Nutritional optic neuropathy*

Table 32-2
Conditions Other Than Alcoholism Associated With Wernicke's Encephalopathy

Any condition associated with persistent vomiting or gastrointestinal disease
   - Hyperemesis gravidarum
   - Pyloric stenosis
   - Esophageal stenosis
   - Bariatric surgery

Any condition associated with starvation
   - Tumors causing anorexia
   - Total parenteral nutrition without B complex vitamins
   - High glucose infusions in patients with nutritional deficiency
   - AIDS
   - Neuropsychiatric conditions
     - Anorexia nervosa
     - Schizophrenia
     - Dementia

Miscellaneous conditions
   - Neonatal illness
   - Hunger strike
   - Prisoners of war
   - Complication of medications

The cause of WE is a deficiency of vitamin B_1 (thiamine), which is a key coenzyme at 3 different points in intermediate carbohydrate metabolism. Depletion of thiamine and the subsequent stress of a glucose load may result in the relatively abrupt onset of WE. Blood levels of thiamine may be normal even in deficiency states, but blood transketolase levels reflect low thiamine levels more accurately. In your patient, however, you should not await the results of blood tests to initiate treatment. In addition, you should obtain serum magnesium levels (magnesium is a cofactor in glycolysis, which utilizes thiamine). If magnesium is low, it should be replaced when treating patients with WE. Thiamine given in a patient with WE, when the magnesium level is low, will fail to reverse the clinical features of WE.

As far as neuroimaging in your patient, I have found computed tomography (CT) studies to be of no help. Magnetic resonance imaging (MRI) in patients with WE reveals a number of lesions best seen on fluid-attenuated inversion recovery (FLAIR), T-2, and diffusion weighted imagaing (DWI) sequences. High signals are found in medial thalamus, the hypothalamus, the mamillary bodies, the periaqueductal region, and surrounding the fourth ventricle. Other areas include the basal ganglia, cerebral cortex, pons, and medulla. Imaging after treatment frequently shows generalized atrophy and volume loss throughout the entire brain.

Your patient should receive the immediate administration of intravenous (IV) thiamine; 100 mg and Mg SO_4 if serum levels are low. Oral thiamine, 50 mg daily, should be administered thereafter. Much has been written about the potential for an anaphylactic reaction to IV thiamine, but I have personally never seen any untoward side effect from IV thiamine. A large study that reviewed the issue of thiamine use and anaphylaxis concluded that the damage due to failure to administer thiamine far outweighed any potential side effects of treatment. Patients with anorexia, severe weight loss of any cause, persistent vomiting, starvation of any cause, and patients who are desperately ill in intensive care settings are, in my experience, all at risk for development of WE.

Summary

* The diagnosis of WE should be considered in any individual who is confused, ataxic, or unable to walk and who has ocular motor or visual problems in the setting of nutritional deficiency of whatever cause.

* Patients with possible WE should have immediate administration of thiamine in doses of 50 to 100 mg that should be given in advance of any IV glucose solutions. Ocular motility should improve within hours. If not, a repeat IV dose of 100 mg thiamine and a large 500 mg oral dose of thiamine should be administered.

* The clinical recovery from WE is uneven. Ocular motor signs improve first and most rapidly. Gait problems may persist due to concomitant nutritional neuropathy and/ or cerebellar degeneration. The full-blown amnestic syndrome recovers fully in less than 20% of patients.

Bibliography

Cain D, Halliday GM, Kril JJ, Harper CG. Operational criteria for the classification of chronic alcoholics: identification of Wernicke's encephalopathy. *J Neurol Neurosurg Psychiatry.* 1997;62:51-60.

Foster D, Falah M, Kadom N, Mandler R. Wernicke encephalopathy after bariatric surgery: losing more than just weight. *Neurology.* 2005;65:1987.

Harper CG, Giles M, Finlay-Jones R. Clinical signs in the Wernicke Korsakoff complex: a retrospection analysis of 131 patients diagnosed at necropsy. *J Neurol Neurosurg Psychiatry.* 1986;49:341-345.

Victor M, Adams KS, Collins GH. *The Wernicke-Korsakoff Syndrome and Related Neurologic Disorders Due to Alcoholism and Malnutrition.* 2nd ed. Philadelphia, PA: FA Davis; 1989.

White ML, Zhang Y, Lee AG, et al. MRI imagining with diffusion weighted imaging in acute and chronic Wernicke encephalopathy. *AJNR.* 2005;26:2306-2310.

33

How Do You Manage Postoperative Visual Loss After Spinal Surgery?

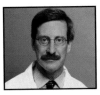

Wayne T. Cornblath, MD

A 45-year-old man who awoke after a lumbar laminectomy blind in both eyes is being examined. What etiologies should be considered? Should steroids be given? Should this patient be transfused?

While your case is that of a patient who had lumbar spinal surgery, postoperative visual loss can occur with virtually any type of surgery. Others reported coronary artery bypass grafting, gastrointestinal, and genitourinary surgeries. In the early 1990s, a number of case reports appeared of postoperative visual loss with spine surgery, as in this case, leading to study and recommendations by the American Society of Anesthesiologists (see below). Discovery of visual complaints can be delayed by the effects of postoperative medications and anesthesia upon the patient sensorium. The exam is more difficult because of the limited conditions under which it is performed (ie, in a hospital room, intensive care unit [ICU], or recovery room) and effect of medications on the exam (ie, miotic pupils and limited cooperation). Finally, medicolegal concerns always seem to arise in a patient who has a potentially devastating complication far from the operative site.

When evaluating postoperative visual loss, the critical decision points are localization, etiology, and treatment. The 5 major possible causes of to be considered are external orbital compression with central retinal artery occlusion (CRAO), ischemic optic neuropathy (anterior or posterior), compression of the optic nerve or chiasm by a pituitary tumor (eg, apoplexy), cortical visual loss, and functional visual loss. The visual involvement can be unilateral or bilateral, mild or severe.

The examination is critical but often difficult. Visual acuity, usually done at near with appropriate presbyopic correction, pupillary testing, confrontation visual fields, external examination, ocular motility, and dilated fundus evaluation are all required.

Orbital compression occurs inadvertently with surgery in the prone position and is usually monocular, associated with ocular motility abnormalities, external edema, chemosis, and fundus findings of central retinal artery occlusion. Visual acuity and visual field function vary greatly.

Ischemic optic neuropathy (ION) will show an afferent pupillary defect if unilateral or bilateral and asymmetric. If bilateral and symmetric, sluggish, poorly reactive pupils are seen. Unfortunately, medications can produce small, poorly reactive pupils and limit evaluation of the pupils. The optic nerves are swollen in roughly half of patients (anterior ION) and normal in the other half (posterior ION). Occasionally, one nerve will be swollen and one nerve normal in patients with bilateral involvement. As in patients with non-arteritic anterior ION, acuity can range from normal to no light perception (NLP) and the typical visual field defect is altitudinal in nature.

Optic neuropathy from an intracranial compressive lesion can be unilateral or bilateral. An afferent pupillary defect will be seen if unilateral or bilateral and asymmetric. Visual acuity can be variable and the typical visual field defect is altitudinal. Typically, there is no optic nerve swelling and and neuroimaging is essential.

Compression of the chiasm will produce variable acuity loss. The visual field findings are the key to this diagnosis with either bitemporal or junctional visual field loss. Typically, the optic nerves are not swollen and again neuroimaging is mandatory.

Cortical visual loss will have 2 patterns. If there is unilateral involvement of the post-chiasmal optic pathway, the patient will have a homonymous hemianopic visual field defect with normal acuity. If there is bilateral involvement of the postchiasmal optic pathways, then bilateral homonymous hemianopic visual field defects with variable loss of acuity will be seen. Macular sparing can leave markedly restricted visual fields with normal visual acuity or there can be variable loss of visual acuity. However, if visual acuity is affected with cortical visual loss, the visual acuity will be identical in each eye. In cortical visual loss, even if the patient is completely blind, the pupils will be normally reactive and the funduscopic appearance will be normal.

Patients with functional visual loss will have inconsistent findings on examination, normal imaging, and at times an indifference to their level of visual loss.

Neuroimaging is critical to confirm a diagnosis of cortical visual loss and in the patient with retrobulbar optic neuropathy or a chiasmal pattern of visual loss to rule out an acute compressive process, typically pituitary apoplexy. Magnetic resonance imaging (MRI) is the preferred imaging modality because of the early detection of infarction, ability to distinguish posterior reversible encephalopathy syndrome (PRES), and superior optic nerve and chiasm imaging (Figure 33-1).

Laboratory evaluation should include hemoglobin to assess for anemia. Checking erythrocyte sedimentation rate (ESR) is not typically helpful as the ESR is routinely elevated postoperatively. Cortisol and thyroid-stimulating hormone (TSH) should be checked if pituitary apoplexy is a consideration.

Treatment of postoperative visual loss is controversial with no clear evidence to guide us. In patients with optic neuropathy and no medical contraindications I recommend transfusion to a hemoglobin of 10 if the patient is below this level. Maintenance of normal

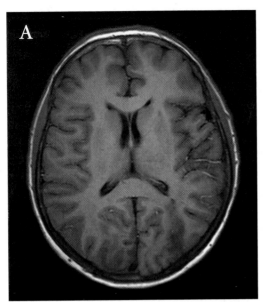 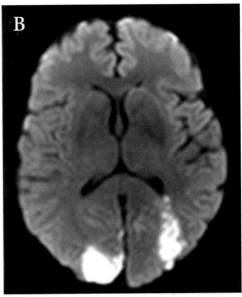

Figure 33-1. (A) Normal T1 MRI in patient with bilateral inferior quadrantanopia on examination. (B) Diffusion weighted imaging shows bilateral occipital infarctions from reversible cerebral vasoconstriction syndrome (Call-Fleming syndrome).

blood pressure and supplemental oxygen are unproven but are additional considerations. I do not believe that there is any proven role for corticosteroid treatment, either high-dose intravenous or oral, intraocular pressure-lowering agents, or antiplatelet medications. Blood pressure and systemic medications (eg, tacrolimus, cyclosporine) must be considered in a patient with PRES. Recovery over time has occurred but is quite variable and impossible to predict.

The American Society of Anesthesiologists has reviewed the topic and published both a practice advisory concerning spine surgery and postoperative visual loss and the results of a retrospective case collection. Risk factors for development of postoperative visual loss include pre-existing vascular risk factors, preoperative anemia, lengthy procedures (9.8 hours ± 3 hours), and significant blood loss (median 2 L, range 0.1 to 25 L). Some authors maintain that intraoperative hypotension is also a factor. Whether these findings apply to other surgeries is not known.

Summary

* The etiology of postoperative ION remains controversial but hypotension and anemia may be associated risk factors.

* There is no proven treatment for postoperative ION.

* Identification of at-risk patients and appropriate informed consent should be considered.

Bibliography

American Society of Anesthesiologists Task Force on Perioperative Blindness. Practice advisory for perioperative visual loss associated with spine surgery: a report by the American Society of Anesthesiologists Task Force on Perioperative Blindness. *Anesthesiology.* 2006;104:1319-1328.

American Society of Anesthesiologists Task Force on Perioperative Blindness. Practice guidelines for perioperative blood transfusion and adjuvant therapies: an updated report by the American Society of Anesthesiologists Task Force on Perioperative Blood Transfusion and Adjuvant Therapies. *Anesthesiology.* 2006;105:198-208.

Buono LM, Foroozan R. Perioperative posterior ischemic optic neuropathy: review of the literature. *Surv Ophthalmol.* 2005;50:15-26.

How Do I Manage Transient Monocular Visual Loss in a Young, Otherwise Healthy Patient?

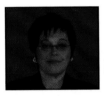

Rosa Ana Tang, MD, MPH

A 27-year-old woman reports having had 3 episodes of transient "darkening" of vision in her right eye. Each episode lasted 3 to 5 minutes without any associated symptoms. Her general health is excellent; her only medication is oral contraceptives. She has no history of migraine. Her examination, including visual fields, is entirely normal. What evaluation and therapy should be undertaken?

Transient monocular vision loss (TMVL) of abrupt onset typically represents a focal retinal, choroidal, or optic nerve functional deficit due to ischemia to the eye. Historical clues are important such as asking your patient what area of the visual field was lost; duration; and presence of any neurological symptom such as headache, numbness, or weakness. In your particular patient the absence of scintillations and headaches and the fact that the vision loss is monocular makes a diagnosis of migraine less likely. A careful history asking for associated systemic symptoms is important, although there are none in your patient.

The differential diagnosis of TMVL in young individuals includes a number of entities. "Vasospasm" in the eye is thought to be due to spasm involving the retinal circulation and often affects the same eye every time. These patients have a stereotypic pattern of "patchy darkening" of vision for approximately 1 minute followed by poor acuity for 1 to 5 minutes with return to baseline vision. There are no scintillations and no neurological abnormalities on examination. In my opinion, the best "investigation" is a thorough neuro-ophthalmology history and exam. I have also found that the frequency of the TMVL events can sometimes be reduced by the use of calcium channel blockers.

Vasospasm has previously been known as retinal migraine, a term still used by some. It is a benign condition that very rarely leads to any permanent visual damage.

Blood abnormalities such as hypercoagulable/hyperviscosity syndromes are also a consideration. The patient in question is taking birth control pills and if she is a smoker and also has history of migraine, she falls in the category of the triple "threat" for stroke risk.

In other cases involving intermittent systemic blood pressure changes (too high or too low), TMVL may be associated with changes in posture, bright light exposure, heavy exercise, or eating a large meal. If paroxysmal hypertension related to renal artery stenosis or pheochromocytoma is the cause, the patient may also experience episodic dizziness as well as palpitations, sweating, and pallor. Cardiac emboli or arrhythmia related to valvular disease such as patent foramen ovale or endocarditis in drug addicts is characterized by erratic pulse and/or heart murmur on physical examination.

Less likely is the presence of premature atherosclerosis, carotid dissection, or fibromuscular dysplasia in which case the patient may have an ipsilateral Horner syndrome. These young patients are unlikely to have significant occlusive carotid artery disease. Other rare causes of TMVL are orbital tumors and posterior vitreous detachment. The latter gives rise to a typical "one time event" of monocular TMVL in the majority of those patients affected. Ocular coherence tomography (OCT) is the instrument of choice to study vitreo-retinal interface and will image the presence of vitreo-retinal traction in these patients.

A standard algorithm for assessment of young patients (<50 years old) with TMVL does not exist and diagnostic evaluation is influenced by the history and specific examination findings such as ocular inflammation, retinal venous or arterial changes, presence of a carotid bruit, level of blood pressure, pulse, heart murmurs, and any neurologic deficits. The importance of a very thorough eye exam is essential, especially dilated funduscopy and visual field testing.

In a healthy young patient with an isolated single episode of TMVL and no other associated symptoms and signs, I would conclude this is due to retinal "vasospasm" and not work-up the patient further. Both visual and systemic prognoses are excellent. However, our patient has had 3 occurrences of TMVL and therefore studies to exclude heart disease, vasculitis, and possibly a hypercoagulable state could be considered (Table 34-1). If all studies are normal, I would reassure the patient of the benign nature of the disorder, and treatment with a calcium channel blocker may be offered. If the patient experiences a change in these stereotypic visual events or new signs and symptoms develop, patient re-evaluation is indicated.

Summary

* Many otherwise healthy young patients with an isolated single episode of TMVL and no other associated symptoms and signs have retinal "vasospasm."

* Selected patients might require testing to exclude heart disease, vasculitis, and possibly a hypercoagulable state.

* A dramatic change in prior stable and stereotypic visual events or the development of new neurologic signs or symptoms should prompt re-evaluation as indicated.

Table 34-1
Hypercoagulable State Testing

- Anticardiolipin (aCL) (IgG or IgM) in serum or plasma
- Phospholipid units (GPL)/mL or IgM phospholipid units (MPL)/mL
- Lupus anticoagulant levels
- Anti–beta-2 glycoprotein I antibodies (IgG or IgM) in serum or plasma
- Homocysteine levels
- Prothrombin fragment 1 and 2
- D-dimer test
- Antithrombin III
- Fibrin and fibrinogen degradation products
- Fibrinopeptide A
- Platelet count
- Fibrinogen
- Prothrombin time
- Activated partial thromboplastin time
- Thrombin time
- INR
- Protamine test
- Factor V
- Protein C and S
- LA in plasma

INR = international normalized ratio; Factor V Leiden; Lupus anticoagulant = LA in plasma

Bibliography

Bernard GA, Bennett JL. Vasospastic amaurosis fugax. *Arch Ophthalmol.* 1999;117:1568-1569.

Booy R. Amaurosis in young women. *Lancet.* 1990;335:1538.

Bousser MG. Migraine, female hormones, and stroke. *Cephalgia.* 1999;19:75-79.

Burger, SK, Saul, RF, Selhorst, JB, et al. Transient monocular blindness caused by vasospasm. *N Engl J Med.* 1991; 325:870-873.

Donders RCJM, Kappelle LJ, Derksen RHWM, et al. Transient monocular blindness and antiphospholipid antibodies in systemic lupus erythematosus. *Neurology.* 1998;51:535-540.

Hoyt WF. Transient monocular visual loss: a historical perspective. *Ophthalmol Clin North Am.* 1996;9:323-325.

O' Sullivan E, Shaunak S, Matthews T, et al. Transient monocular blindness. *J Neurol Neurosurg Psychiatry.* 1995; 59:559.

O' Sullivan E, Rossor M, Elston JS. Amaurosis fugax in young people. *Br J Ophthalmol.* 1992;76:660-662.

Winterkorn JMS, Kupersmith MJ, Wirtschafter JD, et al. Brief report: treatment of vasospastic amaurosis fugax with calcium channel blockers. *N Engl J Med.* 1993;329:396-398.

35

WHAT IS THE EVALUATION FOR TRANSIENT MONOCULAR VISUAL LOSS IN AN OLDER ADULT?

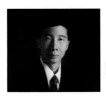

Byron L. Lam, MD

A 72-year-old man who has experienced loss of vision lasting approximately 5 minutes in his left eye 2 days previously is being examined. He had no accompanying symptoms. His review of systems documented a 20-year history of hypertension, and he had coronary artery surgery 2 years ago. Medications include antihypertensives and aspirin. Ophthalmologic evaluation is unremarkable with the exception of a shiny, refractile retinal embolus seen in the left fundus. What should be done next?

I would start by emphasizing the necessity of comprehensive patient evaluation in any older patient with transient monocular visual loss (TMVL). The need for an aggressive evaluation of your patient is even more compelling given the finding of a retinal embolus. I would outline the appropriate diagnostic steps that should be done in establishing a source of retinal emboli and try to define the patient's morbidity and possible mortality following carotid endarterectomy.

Ischemia is the main concern. In older patients with TMVL, carotid artery stenosis, carotid or cardiac embolic phenomenon, and ischemia associated with giant cell arteritis are serious conditions that could potentially not only cause permanent visual loss from ocular ischemia but also increase the risk of morbidity and mortality from cerebral infarction. Therefore, further work-up in an older patient with TMVL is mandatory.

In general, the assessment begins with asking the patient whether the TMVL is complete or partial as well as the duration and frequency of each episode. Typically, these ischemic events last from seconds to several minutes and resolve spontaneously. Patients with partial visual loss related to ischemia are likely to report visual loss to the upper or lower half of the visual field with demarcation between the seeing and non-seeing areas. Increase in frequency of TMVL is particularly worrisome and suggests an increased risk of a permanent ischemic event. Elderly patients with amaurosis should be asked for the presence of giant cell arteritis symptoms, and this should be followed by a work-up for giant cell arteritis if indicated. For all patients with monocular visual loss, a careful past medical history should be obtained with a focus on vascular risk factors including hypertension, diabetes, hyperlipidemia, coronary arterial disease, cardiac arrhythmia, and carotid artery disease. Other factors such as tobacco use and oral contraceptive use may also contribute to the risk of ischemic events. A careful funduscopic examination after pupillary dilation should be performed with an emphasis on detecting retinal intra-arteriolar plaques, an important clinical sign of emboli. The 3 common retinal emboli are cholesterol, platelet-fibrin, and calcific. Cholesterol emboli, also called Hollenhorst plaques, are beige, refractile emboli often found at retinal arteriole bifurcations. Cholesterol emboli are related to atheromatous carotid artery plaques while platelet-fibrin and calcific emboli are associated with thrombus in the carotid artery or from cardiac valves.

For your patient with a visible retinal cholesterol embolus, hypertension, and cardiac arterial disease, I would first check his blood pressure. If the hypertension is poorly controlled (eg, diastolic >100 mmHg), then the patient should be sent promptly to his internist or an urgent care clinic for treatment. The presence of a retinal cholesterol embolus is strongly associated with carotid artery stenosis. I prefer to initiate the work-up by sending the patient for expedited carotid duplex ultrasonogram and it has been my practice to order brain magnetic resonance imaging (MRI) (with and without gadolinium). The carotid duplex is an important test to assess the presence of carotid artery stenosis and atheromatous plaques. The brain MRI will detect whether there are any cerebral infarcts, and the extent of white matter changes on fluid-attenuated inversion recovery (FLAIR) images is an indicator of the degree of arteriosclerosis. If new hemorrhagic infarcts are found, prompt hospital admission by an internist or a stroke specialist should be considered. Other diagnostic considerations include an electrocardiogram to determine the presence of previous myocardial infarction and an echocardiogram to assess any source of cardiac emboli, although this is less likely to produce cholesterol plaques. Clinical applications of newer modalities such as magnetic resonance angiography (MRA) and computed tomography angiography (CTA) are being defined.

You might also be interested in the North American Symptomatic Carotid Endarterectomy Trial (NASCET). This study found carotid endarterectomy to be beneficial in symptomatic patients with 70% or greater stenosis, but carotid endarterectomy is contraindicated if the carotid artery is completely occluded. Ipsilateral stroke in 2 years was 9% in those who had surgery versus 26% in those treated medically. The benefit was significantly reduced for symptomatic patients with less than 50% stenosis. The benefit of surgery in asymptomatic patients with 60% or greater stenosis was significantly less than symptomatic patients with 70% or greater stenosis. For patients who experienced transient monocular visual loss, 6 factors were found to increase the risk of stroke: 1) age >75 years, 2) male sex, 3) history of hemispheric transient ischemic attack or stroke, 4) intermittent claudication, 5) 80% to 94% internal carotid artery stenosis, and 6) no collateral circulation on cerebral angiography. Carotid endarterectomy is likely to be helpful in patients with TMVL when 2 or more of the risk factors are present.

Of interest, in the Asymptomatic Carotid Atherosclerosis Study (ACAS), the 5-year risk for ipsilateral stroke was 5% in those who had surgery compared to 11% for those treated medically. Taken together, consideration for carotid endarterectomy is warranted in symptomatic patients with greater than 50% stenosis (especially in those with 70% or greater stenosis) and healthy asymptomatic patients with greater than 60% stenosis. Also taken into consideration are the facts that perioperative mortality of carotid endarterectomy is in the range of 1% to 2% and postoperative strokes occur in 1% to 5% of patients. In addition, if carotid endarterectomy is considered after carotid duplex testing, additional imaging of the carotid bifurcation is indicated. Currently, this varies with the medical faculty involved but should include MRA, CTA, and/or catheter (digital subtraction) angiography.

The visual prognosis of patients experiencing TMVL is generally favorable and is related to the extent of carotid stenosis and the frequency of recurrent emboli. Mortality is increased in patients with TMVL, and death has been found to be more likely to result from myocardial infarction than from stroke. When pooled data from 2 population studies, the Beaver Dam Eye Study and the Blue Mountains Eye Study, were analyzed, the presence of retinal arteriolar emboli increased all-cause mortality by approximately 30% over 10 to 12 years.

Newer surgical alternatives to carotid endarterectomy include angioplasty and stenting, and investigations are continuing to define their clinical applications. These alternatives warrant consideration, particularly in patients at high risk for carotid endarterectomy. However, the risks and benefits of these newer procedures compared to carotid endarterectomy are not yet clarified based on recent clinical trials (SAPPHIRE, EVA-3S, and SPACE trials).

Medical treatments in patients with carotid stenosis and emboli include antiplatelet agents such as aspirin and clopidogrel (Plavix [Bristol-Myers Squibb/Sanofi Pharmaceuticals Partnership, Bridgewater, NJ]). Ticlopidine (Ticlid [Roche Laboratory Inc, Nutley, NJ]) is used less often because of the risk of neutropenia. In this patient who is already on aspirin, the addition of clopidogrel can be considered. Anticoagulation using warfarin in patients with non-cardiac emboli is controversial.

Summary

* Work-up in older patients with TMVL with a visible acute and symptomatic retinal cholesterol embolus is recommended.

* Referral to a neuro-ophthalmologist, internist, or stroke specialist for further work-up might be indicated.

* A careful history and examination by the ophthalmologist can help to triage the urgency of the evaluation and direct the evaluation.

Bibliography

Barnett HJ, Taylor DW, Eliasziw M, et al. Benefit of carotid endarterectomy in patients with symptomatic moderate or severe stenosis. North American Symptomatic Carotid Endarterectomy Trial Collaborators. *N Engl J Med.* 1998;339:1415-1425.

Executive Committee for the Asymptomatic Carotid Atherosclerosis Study. Endarterectomy for asymptomatic carotid artery stenosis. *JAMA.* 1995;273:1421-1428.

Inzitari D, Eliasziw M, Gates P, et al. The causes and risk of stroke in patients with asymptomatic internal-carotid-artery stenosis. North American Symptomatic Carotid Endarterectomy Trial Collaborators. *N Engl J Med.* 2000;342:1693-1700.

Mas JL, Chatellier G, Beyssen B, et al. Endarterectomy versus stenting in patients with symptomatic severe carotid stenosis. *N Engl J Med.* 2006;355:1660-1671.

North American Symptomatic Carotid Endarterectomy Trial Collaborators. Beneficial effect of carotid endarterectomy in symptomatic patients with high-grade carotid stenosis. *N Engl J Med.* 1991;325:445-453.

The SPACE Collaborative Group. 30 day results from the SPACE trial of stent-protected angioplasty versus carotid endarterectomy in symptomatic patients: a randomized non-inferiority trial. *Lancet.* 2006;368:1239-1247.

Wang JJ, Cugati S, Knudtson MD, et al. Retinal arteriolar emboli and long-term mortality: pooled data analysis from two older populations. *Stroke.* 2006;37:1833-1836.

Yadav JS, Wholey MH, Kuntz RE, et al. Protected carotid-artery stenting versus endarterectomy in high-risk patients. *N Engl J Med.* 2004;351:1493-1501.

WHAT IS THE EVALUATION FOR A HOMONYMOUS HEMIANOPIA?

Jonathan C. Horton, MD, PhD

A 67-year-old man developed visual loss. His visual field shows a right homonymous hemiano-
pia. Are there characteristics of the field defect or any associated symptoms that might provide a
clue as to the localization of the lesion? What type of imaging study should be performed and how
urgently should it be done? Is there any proven treatment for homonymous visual field defects?

Homonymous hemianopia refers to a field defect caused by a lesion of the visual
system posterior to the optic chiasm. When discovered as an acute finding, as in your
patient, it is a sign of serious intracranial disease that requires emergency evaluation.

The decussation of nasal retinal fibers at the optic chiasm unites in the visual
pathway each eye's representation of the contralateral hemifield of vision (Figure
36-1). Consequently, damage to the optic tract, lateral geniculate nucleus, optic radiations, or visual cortex produces an overlapping pattern of visual field loss in each
eye, which usually respects the vertical meridian. Patients are sometimes unaware
of a fresh hemianopia or erroneously attribute their symptoms to monocular visual
loss. Careful testing of the visual fields is the crux of accurate diagnosis. Perimetry
should be obtained in any patient complaining of unexplained visual loss. My preference is the Humphrey 24-2 SITA program (Carl Zeiss Meditec, Jena, Germany)
because it provides threshold data in only a few minutes per eye. Although it does
not test the peripheral field, the risk of missing a hemianopia is small because the
representation of the central field is highly magnified in the brain. In fact, the central
24 degrees occupy 70% of the postchiasmal visual pathway. If computerized perimetry is

Figure 36-1. Diagram of the visual pathway. The postchiasmal regions where a lesion will produce a contralateral homonymous hemianopia are highlighted in red.

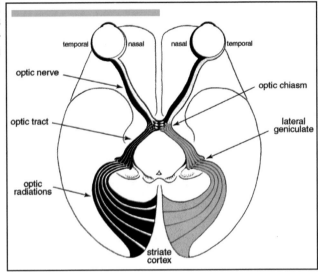

not available immediately, the visual fields should be tested manually, at least by finger confrontation.

Hemianopia is usually incomplete; the amount of similarity between the pattern of visual field loss in each eye is referred to as the "congruity." The degree of congruity is not a reliable criterion for localizing the site of pathology, perhaps because many lesions involve both the optic radiations and visual cortex. In any case, localization based on exam findings is moot because all patients with hemianopia require neuroimaging. I would refer this patient to the hospital for urgent brain scanning and inpatient neurological evaluation.

Any process that can injure the brain can give rise to a homonymous hemianopia (Table 36-1). The most common etiology is stroke. It can be caused by hemorrhage, embolus, thrombosis, dissection, or vasculitis. In patients with stroke involving the middle cerebral territory, there are often accompanying signs, such as hemiplegia, hemianesthesia, dysphasia, or stupor. In contrast, patients with stroke from involvement of the posterior cerebral artery may have no findings except for hemianopia. In this setting, the diagnosis can be missed by the ophthalmologist who neglects visual field testing. Sometimes the patient may report an episode of acute vertigo, numbness, or diplopia, suggesting an embolus that has become lodged in a posterior cerebral artery after traveling up the basilar artery.

Patients who are evaluated within 3 hours of the onset of symptoms may be candidates for treatment with intravenous tissue plasminogen activator. In practice, few patients with isolated hemianopia receive medical care within this time frame because they do not realize the seriousness of their predicament. Nonetheless, urgent neurologic evaluation is still advisable to reduce the likelihood of stroke progression or occurrence of a second event. In fact, even if hemianopia is not present on an office exam, a reliable history of a transient ischemic attack that produced temporary hemianopic visual loss should trigger prompt referral.

What type of imaging study should be obtained? Noncontrast computerized tomography is low cost, rapid, and available in any emergency room. It is excellent for exclusion

Table 36-1

Causes of Homonymous Hemianopia*

- Stroke (embolic, thrombotic, hemorrhagic, vasculitic, dissection)
- Tumor (primary or metastasis)
- Trauma
- Infection (bacterial, fungal, viral, parasitic)
- Arteriovenous malformation
- Nonorganic visual loss
- Demyelination
- Migraine
- Congenital malformation
- Perinatal hypoxic or hemorrhagic injury
- Posterior reversible leukoencephalopathy
- Neurosurgery; occipital lobe retraction syndrome
- Eclampsia
- Dementia
- Epilepsy
- Mitochondrial myopathy, encephalopathy, lactic acidosis, and stroke (MELAS)
- Drug toxicity (cyclosporine, tacrolimus, sirolimus)
- Nonketotic hyperglycemia

*Stroke, tumor, and trauma account for more than 95% of cases.

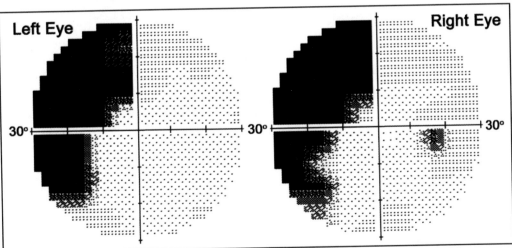

Figure 36-2. Left homonymous hemianopia, mapped with a Humphrey threshold program, showing macular sparing, as well as partial sparing of the lower visual field.

of hemorrhagic stroke and especially suitable in the setting of head trauma. However, magnetic resonance imaging (MRI) is more sensitive for the detection of nonhemorrhagic ischemia from stroke, as well as identification of other lesions such as demyelinating plaques, tumors, and infections. Figure 36-2 shows the visual fields from a patient who reported a 10-day history of a shadow in her vision on the left side. Computed tomography revealed no abnormality. Regular T2-weighted MRI sequences were also near normal

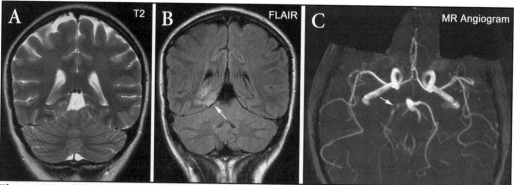

Figure 36-3. (A) Coronal T2-weighted MR scan from the patient with the partial left homonymous hemianopia illustrated in Figure 36-2. The study appears virtually normal. (B) MR FLAIR image showing an ischemic stroke (arrow) involving the lower bank of the calcarine fissure, where the upper quadrant of the visual field is represented in the primary (striate) visual cortex. (C) MR angiogram showing partial occlusion (arrow) of the right posterior cerebral artery, presumably from an embolus.

(Figure 36-3A). However, fluid-attenuated inversion recovery (FLAIR) sequences showed an infarct involving the lower, right calcarine visual cortex in the territory of the lingual artery (Figure 36-3B). MR angiography showed partial occlusion of the proximal right posterior cerebral artery (Figure 36-3C). Another advantage of MRI is that fresh infarcts can be detected sooner than by computed tomography. Diffusion-weighted MRI demonstrates cytotoxic edema within 30 minutes of stroke onset. Computed tomography, as well as standard T1 and T2 MRI sequences, require many hours before any abnormality becomes visible.

If noncontrast studies show no evidence of stroke, gadolinium should be administered to the patient. It increases the sensitivity of MRI for the detection of tumors and infections. Once the etiology of the homonymous hemianopia is established through review of the patient's history, findings, and neuroimaging studies, a focused laboratory evaluation is appropriate. A stroke work-up usually includes echocardiography, vascular imaging, outpatient electrocardiographic monitoring, and selected hematological studies. For tumor, a biopsy is usually performed. Removal of a solitary metastasis may be advisable, depending on the patient's overall prognosis.

The prognosis for homonymous hemianopia depends on its etiology. For a few months after trauma or stroke, improvement can occur spontaneously, especially in patients with an incomplete hemianopia. Surgery for a tumor, arteriovenous malformation, or infectious lesion sometimes worsens a hemianopia by damaging surrounding brain tissue. Occasional patients with homonymous hemianopia have macular sparing, usually from collateral blood flow via the middle cerebral artery to the occipital pole, where central vision is represented. These individuals are able to read normally and adapt better to their handicap than patients with macular splitting. Unfortunately, rehabilitation strategies for patients with hemianopia based on prisms, visual exercises, or computer training are not effective. Patients with a complete hemianopia must be told explicitly by the ophthalmologist that it is not safe or legal to drive. Patients with a partial hemianopia should be retested by the state motor vehicle division to assess their ability to drive.

Summary

* The prognosis for homonymous hemianopia depends on the specific underlying etiology.

* Post-traumatic, hemorrhage-related, or ischemic stroke patients may demonstrate spontaneous improvement over time especially in incomplete hemianopias.

* Surgery for a tumor, arteriovenous malformation, or infectious lesion sometimes worsens a hemianopia by damaging surrounding brain tissue.

* Rehabilitation strategies for patients with homonymous hemianopia may be considered but prisms, visual exercises, or computer training have not been proven to be effective.

Bibliography

Kedar S, Zhang X, Lynn MJ, Newman NJ, Biousse V. Congruency in homonymous hemianopia. *Am J Ophthalmol.* 2007;143:772-780.

Pambakian A, Currie J, Kennard C. Rehabilitation strategies for patients with homonymous visual field defects. *J Neuroophthalmol.* 2005;25:136-142.

van der Worp HB, van Gijn J. Clinical practice: acute ischemic stroke. *N Engl J Med.* 2007;357:572-579.

Zhang X, Kedar S, Lynn MJ, Newman NJ, Biousse V. Homonymous hemianopias: clinical-anatomic correlations in 904 cases. *Neurology.* 2006;66:906-910.

WHAT IS THE EVALUATION FOR A PUPIL-INVOLVED THIRD NERVE PALSY?

Sang-Rog Oh, MD
(co-authored with Gautam R. Mirchandani, MD
and Jeffrey Odel, MD)

A 38-year-old man presents with a complete left third nerve palsy. The left pupil is 7 mm and nonreactive and the right pupil is 3 mm and reactive to light. The patient reports increasing headaches but has no other systemic complaints. He takes no medications regularly and denies a previous history of any double vision. What should be done with his evaluation?

In an isolated third nerve palsy, you should first determine the function of the pupil and the extent of the involvement of the extraocular muscles. As you know, the third cranial nerve innervates the levator palpebrae superioris, superior rectus, medial rectus, inferior rectus, and inferior oblique muscles. The parasympathetic fibers to the pupillary sphincter and ciliary muscles also travel within the nerve. As it makes its way from the brainstem to the orbit, the third nerve may be affected anywhere along its course. According to the "rule of the pupil," if the pupil is dilated and sluggish or nonreactive to light, the presence of an aneurysm must be ruled out. Because the pupillary fibers are located on the dorsal medial surface of the third nerve in the subarachnoid space, a compressive lesion will often affect the pupil first. On the other hand, if the pupil is spared, microvascular ischemia, frequently associated with diabetes mellitus or systemic hypertension, is most likely responsible. You should remember, however, that the rule of the pupil is only applicable in situations where *all* the muscles innervated by the third nerve are impaired and where the palsy is isolated (ie, there are no other neurologic deficits present). Moreover, the rule may not hold true if the pupil is only partially affected and must be applied with caution in young patients.

Figure 37-1. Conventional catheter angiogram clearly demonstrates a right posterior communicating artery (PCoA) aneurysm in a 45-year-old patient who presented with an isolated right third nerve palsy. The aneurysm (arrow) has a narrow neck, measures 6 mm, and is directed posteriorly and inferiorly.

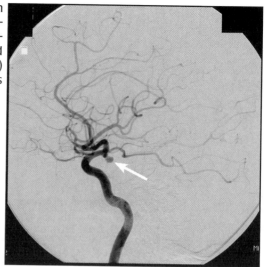

The 2 most frequent causes of an acquired nontraumatic, isolated, and painful third cranial nerve palsy with pupillary involvement in adults are compression from a posterior communicating artery aneurysm (Figure 37-1) and microvascular ischemia of the nerve. An aneurysm must be excluded emergently as intracranial hemorrhage from its rupture may lead to death or severe neurologic morbidity. Pain or ache in and around the eye, orbit, or head does not completely distinguish between these entities as patients with microvascular infarction may complain of some discomfort. Marked neck pain or neck stiffness related to meningismus, however, is highly suggestive of a ruptured aneurysm with subarachnoid blood. A substantial percentage of cases of microvascular infarction will have some pupillary involvement, perhaps up to 30%, though classically it tends to spare the pupil. In contrast, an isolated third nerve palsy with complete paresis of all the muscles innervated by the third nerve and absolute sparing of the pupil is almost never due to an aneurysm. In your patient, the absence of diabetes or other vascular risk factors does not rule out microvascular infarction and the mere presence of diabetes does not exclude aneurysm.

We would recommend that you first ensure that the palsy is neurologically isolated. Other cranial nerve involvement must be eliminated to accurately localize and establish the need for further work-up. Ipsilateral ocular sympathetic involvement should be ruled out by searching for failure of the pupil to dilate in darkness and persistent ptosis on downgaze, indicating dilator weakness and Müller's muscle weakness. Intact abduction and incyclotorsion on abduction should be checked to rule out ipsilateral sixth and/or fourth nerve involvement. Trigeminal sensation in V1, V2, and V3 should be checked. If any of these signs are present, a posterior communicating artery aneurysm is not likely the cause, but a process in the cavernous sinus and subarachnoid space should be suspected. After checking local cranial nerve function, long tract signs such as strength and reflexes in the extremities, face, and great toe should be examined to rule out a midbrain process. Furthermore, check for tremor and cerebellar signs. A third nerve palsy in the setting of contralateral weakness may be caused by a posterior communicating artery aneurysm pressing against the cerebral peduncle at the origin of the third nerve and requires appropriate work-up, whereas a third nerve palsy with cerebellar dysfunction and tremor is likely due to an infarction, multiple sclerosis, or tumor.

We would recommend that your patient have an emergent imaging study. The issue is which study. Magnetic resonance imaging (MRI) of the brain is our preferred first line imaging study for third nerve pathology and the radiologist should be informed of the possibility of a posterior communicating artery aneurysm. Aneurysm is the likely culprit in our patient, so a magnetic resonance angiography (MRA) or computed tomography angiography (CTA) of the brain should be performed with the MRI. In this setting, MRI is a superior modality owing to its capabilities at both localizing an aneurysm and assessing brain parenchyma for some of the other etiologies described above—infarction, demyelination, or tumor among others. The alternative, however, is that CT may more readily detect a subarachnoid hemorrhage. In a patient with severe headache or signs of subarachnoid hemorrhage, a noncontrast CT scan may be the superior initial study. Thus, the choice of the initial study must be tailored to the individual patient. In addition to demyelination, vascular malformation, mass lesion, or stroke of the brainstem, the scan may also demonstrate a compressive lesion of the peripheral portion of CNIII, such as schwannoma or pituitary tumor.

Recently, MRA and CTA have become first-line studies because they are noninvasive and more readily available. A CTA may be better than an MRA in localizing an aneurysm and it can also identify vascular calcification. MRA does not use ionizing radiation and may be performed during the same evaluation as the initial MRI and MRI is generally superior to CT scan for evaluating nonaneurysmal causes of third nerve palsy. The reliability of a CT/CTA or MRI/MRA depends on the quality of the images, the institution performing the studies, and the skill of the neuroradiologist interpreting them. We have encountered several cases where the initial reading did not show the presence of an aneurysm only to see one later on conventional catheter angiography. With the appropriate techniques, an MRA or CTA will detect 97% of aneurysms larger than 5 mm in diameter, but a significant number of lesions measuring less than 5 mm can still be missed. Although these smaller lesions represent only 10% of aneurysms causing a third nerve palsy, they still carry a risk of rupture and can lead to disastrous consequences.

If the initial studies are equivocal, a conventional catheter angiography should be considered if other etiologies have been ruled out. The disadvantage of catheter angiography is its overall complication rate, reported to be as high as 8%, with permanent neurologic morbidity as high as 2%. Recent improvements in catheter design, technique, and the use of nonionic contrast have significantly decreased the likelihood of adverse events. Nevertheless, the risks of a conventional angiogram must be weighed against the level of suspicion for an aneurysm. We believe, therefore, that in cases where there is a high suspicion of an aneurysm, conventional catheter angiography should still be considered even if the MRI/MRA or CT/CTA is normal.

Summary

* In a patient with a complete, isolated third nerve palsy with pupillary involvement, an aneurysm is the most likely cause.

* MRI with MRA or CTA of the head should be initially performed but a conventional catheter angiography might still be necessary if the suspicion for aneurysm remains high.

Bibliography

Bruce BB, Biousse V, Newman NJ. Third nerve palsies. *Sem Neurol.* 2007;27(3):257-268.

Kassell NF, Torner JC. Size of intracranial aneurysms. *Neurosurgery.* 1983;12:291-297.

Lee AG, Hayman LA, Brazis PW. The evaluation of isolated third nerve palsy revisited: an update on the evolving role of magnetic resonance, computed tomography, and catheter angiography. *Surv Ophthalmol.* 2002; 47(2):137-157.

Trobe JD. Third nerve palsy and the pupil: footnotes to the rule. *Arch Ophthalmol.* 1988;106:601-602.

WHAT IS THE EVALUATION FOR A PAINFUL THIRD NERVE PALSY WITHOUT A FIXED AND DILATED PUPIL BUT WITH ANISOCORIA (PARTIAL PUPIL INVOLVEMENT)?

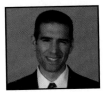

Michael S. Vaphiades, DO

A 67-year-old woman presents with pain and a third nerve palsy OD. Her pupil is slightly bigger on the right side, but the pupil is still reactive.

The management of your patient requires review of the "rule of the pupil." Put simply, the rule states that a compressive lesion of the third nerve (particularly an aneurysm) will cause a fixed, dilated pupil. In contrast, third cranial nerve palsy from an ischemic mononeuropathy (diabetes, hypertension) demonstrates no anisocoria and the pupil is briskly reactive. There are important caveats associated with these guidelines:

* A third cranial nerve palsy due to aneurysmal compression at or near the junction of the internal carotid and posterior communicating arteries may initially demonstrate normal pupillary size and reactivity in 14% of patients, but pupillary involvement may develop in the ensuing 7 to 10 days.

* To be judged "pupil sparing," the isocoric and reactive pupil of the third cranial nerve palsy must be seen in a setting of complete ophthalmoplegia.

* It has been reported that an ischemic third cranial nerve palsy due to diabetes may have anisocoria up to 2.5 mm.

Where does this leave us in evaluating your 67-year-old diabetic woman with a painful third cranial nerve palsy and an enlarged yet reactive pupil? Pain may be present with both compressive and ischemic causes, so this symptom is of limited diagnostic help. One possibility is that your patient may have aneurysmal compression and with careful follow-up she might develop a fixed, dilated pupil. She may also have a diabetic ophthalmoplegia with a slightly dilated pupil that remains reactive.

Because an intracranial aneurysm is a life-threatening condition, I would emergently order a computed tomography angiography (CTA) because I believe that the maximum intensity projection (MIP) images on the CTA are often better than conventional CT scanning. In one study you can get all the information that you need. In either case, if the conventional CT scan is normal, then I would obtain a CTA and if the conventional CT is abnormal (subarachnoid hemorrhage), then I would still order a CTA. I prefer the CTA because it is a low-risk test with good resolution in detecting an aneurysm. On the way to the scanner, since she may also have a vasculopathic process, I would obtain a complete blood count, metabolic panel, cholesterol, and triglycerides to survey for leukopenia, anemia, thrombocytopenia, diabetes, renal failure, and hyperlipidemia—all of which may potentially impact diagnosis and treatment. The creatinine should be done "stat" because the patient must have normal renal function to have a CTA. I would ask about giant cell arteritis symptoms (jaw claudication, scalp tenderness, weight loss, fever/chills, headache, or myalgias) and consider an erythrocyte sedimentation rate and C-reactive protein.

The CTA must be of high quality at an institution skilled with this technology and with radiologists familiar with the software. High-quality CTA may detect intracranial aneurysms as small as 3 mm in size.

If the CTA is normal, then a vasculopathic process is assumed. Vasculopathic risk factors need to be controlled and any lab abnormalities addressed. If platelets are normal and there is no history of gastric ulcers, start one baby (coated) aspirin daily with food.

By 3 months, there should be complete or near complete resolution of the third cranial nerve palsy (rarely longer, but always less than 6 months). If, at this point, there is persistent ophthalmoplegia, other cranial neuropathies develop, or if signs of aberrant regeneration are found, then further imaging studies are warranted. This would include a contrasted, fat-suppressed magnetic resonance imaging (MRI) scan. Some authors might start with MRI and magnetic resonance angiography (MRA) combination and this depends on your local institutional expertise with the various imaging modalities. If in doubt, you should consult with your local neuroradiologist on the best imaging studies at your institution.

If an aneurysm is still suspected, intra-arterial catheter angiography may still be indicated.

I think that the most likely cause of your patient's third cranial nerve palsy is microvascular ischemia and there will be complete resolution of the cranial neuropathy. However, for any patient presenting with a third cranial palsy and any anisocoria, aneurysmal compression must be considered. Such patients require meticulous clinical evaluation and judicious use of neuroimaging studies.

Summary

* The evaluation of patients with a third nerve palsy needs to be individualized.

* If an aneurysm is highly suspected, intra-arterial catheter angiography may still be indicated despite previous negative neuroimaging.

* Microvascular ischemic palsies resolve over time.

Bibliography

Burde RM, Savino PJ, Trobe JD. *Clinical Decisions in Neuro-Ophthalmology.* 3rd ed. St Louis, MO: Mosby; 2002.

El Khaldi M, Pernter P, Ferro F, et al. Detection of cerebral aneurysms in nontraumatic subarachnoid hemorrhage: role of multislice CT angiography in 130 consecutive patients. *Radiol Med.* 2007;112:123-137.

Jacobson DM. Pupil involvement in patients with diabetes-associated oculomotor nerve palsy. *Arch Ophthalmol.* 1998;116:723-727.

Jacobson DM. Relative pupil-sparing third nerve palsy: etiology and clinical variables predictive of a mass. *Neurology.* 2001;56:797-798.

Kissel JT, Burde RM, Klingele TG, Zeiger HE. Pupil-sparing oculomotor palsies with internal carotid-posterior communicating artery aneurysms. *Ann Neurol.* 1983;13:149-154.

Trobe JD. Isolated pupil-sparing third nerve palsy. *Ophthalmology.* 1985;92:58-61.

Trobe JD. Third nerve palsy and the pupil: footnotes to the rule. *Arch Ophthalmol.* 1988;106:601-602.

Trobe JD. Managing oculomotor nerve palsy. *Arch Ophthalmol.* 1998;116:798.

Vaphiades MS, Horton JA. MRA or CTA, that's the question. *Surv Ophthalmol.* 2005;50:406-410.

This chapter is dedicated to Dan Jacobson, whose research provided much of the data used in this chapter. Dan's premature death will curtail neuro-ophthalmologic research for decades to come.

39

HOW DO YOU MANAGE AN ISOLATED AND PRESUMED VASCULOPATHIC PUPIL-SPARING THIRD NERVE PALSY?

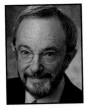

Thomas J. Carlow, MD

An 80-year-old woman presents with a complete left third nerve palsy. Pupils measured 5 mm bilaterally and both reacted normally to light. She had been treated for hypertensive vascular disease for the past 25 years. The patient felt well although did report increasing headaches recently and some decrease in her overall level of energy. What is the appropriate evaluation?

I would first determine if the remainder of her general, ophthalmologic, and neurologic examinations were normal. I will assume that this patient's exam was otherwise unremarkable and that she had no history of trauma.

To begin with, in order to label a third nerve palsy "pupil-sparing," there must be complete ptosis and external ophthalmoplegia yet the pupils are isocoric and react equally well to light and near stimuli. If the ophthalmoplegia and ptosis are only partial, then the status of the pupil remains uncertain. Maximal external ophthalmoplegia in an ischemic third nerve palsy is typically complete within a week from the onset and is frequently preceded by periorbital pain.

The patient's long-standing hypertension would tend to support a vasculopathic or ischemic etiology for her third nerve palsy. A vasculoplastic process is the most frequent cause of an isolated pupil-sparing third nerve palsy and is commonly associated with hypertension, diabetes mellitus, atherosclerosis, vasculitis, hyperlipidemia, smoking, and advanced age. A fasting blood sugar, lipid profile, antinuclear antibody (ANA), and hemoglobin A_{1C} should be considered. A vasculopathic process is a strong possibility in your patient.

Since your patient complained of generalized fatigue, it would be extremely important to determine if her headache is localized to her temples and if that region is tender to the touch, suggesting a diagnosis of giant cell arteritis (GCA). Jaw, tongue, and swallowing claudication; weight loss; fever; transient visual loss; myalgias; and arthralgias would make GCA a definite diagnostic possibility. Third nerve palsy with a normal or dilated pupil can occur with GCA and may be the presenting sign. Ischemia of the extraocular muscles in GCA may also result in an ocular motility disorder mimicking a third nerve palsy. GCA is more common in women and increases with age. Although some might disagree, I personally believe that anyone over age 50 with an isolated ocular motor cranial nerve palsy, including your patient, should have a Westergren erythrocyte sedimentation rate (ESR) and a C-reactive protein (CRP). The combination of both an abnormal ESR and CRP will identify almost all patients with GCA with a higher sensitivity, 99.2%, than will either test run separately. If her history is consistent with the diagnosis of GCA, corticosteroids should be started immediately and a temporal artery biopsy performed urgently. However, not all patients with an elevated ESR and/or CRP have GCA. An increased ESR and/or CRP can be seen in many disorders, including lymphoma, carcinoma, myeloma, renal disease, infection, and collagen vascular disease.

Myasthenia gravis and thyroid eye disease can mimic a pupil-sparing third nerve palsy. An ice test on her ptotic lid, an acetylcholine receptor antibody panel (binding, blocking, and modulating), and thyroid function tests should be considered depending on her history and your clinical suspicion. Systemic lupus erythematosus, lymphoma, leukemia, monoclonal gammopathy, syphilis, and viral inflammation may cause a pupil-sparing third nerve palsy. A complete blood count (CBC), venereal disease research laboratory (VDRL) test, fluorescent treponemal antibody absorbed (FTA-Abs) test, serum protein electrophoresis, and an ANA could also be considered.

The history of when the pupil-sparing third nerve palsy became manifest is extremely important. If the pupil is spared only a day from the onset, especially if the ophthalmoplegia is not totally complete, the patient should be closely monitored, particularly within the first week, and at weekly intervals for the first few weeks to be assured that the pupil remains spared. If the pupil becomes dilated during this period of time, neuroimaging including magnetic resonance imaging (MRI) and computed tomography angiography (CTA) and possibly a cerebral angiogram would be indicated to exclude a compressive lesion, particularly an aneurysm. In addition, a patient with a pupil-sparing third nerve palsy present for 3 months or more without signs of resolution should have an MRI, with and without contrast, and a magnetic resonance angiography (MRA) or preferably a CTA. If she develops subtle anisocoria, greater than 0.5 mm, while being monitored, I would have a low threshold for requesting an MRI, an MRA, or a CTA. Finally, a compressive lesion must be considered should signs of third nerve aberrant regeneration develop and an MRI and a CTA would be in order.

In your patient I would obtain a CBC, fasting blood sugar, hemoglobin A_{1C}, ESR, and CRP. The patient's systemic symptoms coupled with the results of the ESR and CRP may necessitate a temporal artery biopsy. Your patient should be instructed to call immediately if her pupil dilates or if she develops new signs or symptoms. Any atypical features or findings would lower my threshold for obtaining an MRI and a CTA. I would see her back in a week and then again in a month. An MRI and if needed a CTA would be ordered if there were no signs of resolution at 3 months. As she improves, an eye patch or possibly a Fresnel prism could help alleviate her double vision.

I would mention, however, that there is some controversy, as with any difficult diagnostic decision, with this paradigm and some authors would suggest that a neuroimaging study does have a role in the initial evaluation of an acute complete third nerve palsy, even with the pupil spared.

Summary

* Consider checking blood pressure and ordering laboratory studies (eg, CBC, fasting blood sugar, hemoglobin A_{1C}, ESR, and CRP) in patients with a pupil-sparing third nerve palsy.

* The patient should be instructed to call immediately if the initially uninvolved pupil dilates or if there are new signs or symptoms suggestive of an aneurysm.

* Atypical features for ischemic palsy should prompt consideration for obtaining an MRI with MRA or CTA.

Bibliography

Capo H, Warren F, Kupersmith M. Evolution of oculomotor nerve palsies. *J Clin Neuro-Ophthalmol.* 1992;12:21-25.

Chou L, Galetta S, Liu G, et al. Acute ocular motor mononeuropathies: prospective study of the roles of neuroimaging and clinical assessment. *J Neurol Sci.* 2004;219:35-39.

Jacobson D. Relative pupil-sparing third nerve palsy: etiology and clinical variables predictive of a mass. *Neurology.* 2001;56:797-798.

Kupersmith M, Heller G, Cox T. Magnetic resonance angiography and clinical evaluation of third nerve palsies and posterior communicating artery aneurysms. *J Neurosurg.* 2006;105:228-234.

Parikh M, Miller N, Lee A, et al. Prevalence of normal C-reactive protein with an elevated erythrocyte sedimentation rate in biopsy-proven giant cell arteritis. *Ophthalmology.* 2006;113:1842-1845.

Schultz K, Lee A. Diagnostic yield of the evaluation of isolated third nerve palsy in adults. *Can J Ophthalmol.* 2007;42:110-115.

WHAT IS THE APPROPRIATE EVALUATION OF A FOURTH NERVE PALSY?

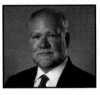

Robert L. Tomsak, MD, PhD
(co-authored with Matthew J. Thurtell, MBBS, FRACP)

A 50-year-old man presents with the complaint that "things seem tilted." He has a left head tilt and binocular vertical diplopia with a right hypertropia. How should I evaluate this patient?

Fourth nerve palsy results in weakness of the superior oblique muscle, which normally depresses and intorts the eye, and thus it can produce both vertical and torsional diplopia. Torsional diplopia, where one image is tilted relative to the other, is especially suggestive of fourth nerve palsy. Asking for a detailed description of the diplopia is therefore the first step in the evaluation of this patient. As patients with fourth nerve palsy often report that their diplopia is increased with downward gaze (eg, while reading) and gaze to the opposite side, you should ask what exacerbates the diplopia with these points in mind. It also helps to ask about the tempo of onset of the diplopia, as this varies depending on the etiology. For example, sudden onset of vertical-torsional diplopia, with or without pain, suggests a microvascular fourth nerve palsy, while gradual onset or intermittent vertical diplopia could be due to decompensation of a long-standing fourth nerve palsy.

We always enquire about a history of head trauma, as this is the most frequently identified cause of fourth nerve palsy. Ask about comorbidities, such as hypertension, diabetes, and other vascular risk factors, as their presence suggests a microvascular etiology in isolated acute-onset fourth nerve palsy. It is also important to ask your patient about any other neurologic symptoms that might help to localize the lesion.

Before assessing extraocular movements, we would note the head position. Tilting of the head to one side, to help minimize diplopia, is a valuable clue to the presence of a fourth nerve palsy on the other side. If there is a head tilt, we ask to inspect old

Figure 40-1. This woman presented with vertical-torsional diplopia and was noted to have a right hypertropia that increased with leftward gaze. (A) The hypertropia was also increased by head tilt to the right, (B) while it was minimized by head tilt to the left, confirming the diagnosis of right fourth nerve palsy.

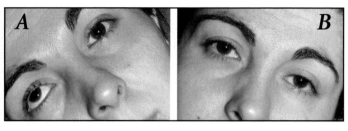

photographs; if a fourth nerve palsy is ultimately diagnosed, the presence of the head tilt in these photographs suggests that the palsy is either congenital or longstanding. After assessing extraocular movements, use the Parks-Bielschowsky 3-step test to confirm the diagnosis of fourth nerve palsy. The first step of this test is to determine the side of the hypertropia. The next step is to show that the hypertropia increases with adduction. The final step is to show that the hypertropia also increases with head tilt to the ipsilateral side (Figure 40-1A). In contrast, the hypertropia will be minimized with head tilt to the contralateral side (Figure 40-1B). In a patient with right hypertropia due to a right fourth nerve palsy, you would therefore expect the vertical deviation to be greatest with leftward gaze and with head tilt to the right. In subtle cases, it may be helpful to quantify the deviation at each stage of the test using vertical prisms or the Maddox rod. Prisms can also be used to demonstrate an increased vertical fusion amplitude (of more than 10 prism diopters), a finding that is often associated with long-standing fourth nerve palsy. Excyclotorsion of the affected eye can be demonstrated and quantified with double Maddox rods. Alternatively, use of Lancaster red-green glasses or examination of the fundus may confirm that the eye is excyclotorted.

Many patients with fourth nerve palsy due to head trauma actually have bilateral fourth nerve palsies. They will usually have hypertropia of each eye on adduction and the Parks-Bielschowsky test might be positive bilaterally. A measured torsional misalignment of more than 8 degrees on double Maddox rod testing is particularly suggestive of bilateral fourth nerve palsies.

During the examination, we would look for signs that help to localize the lesion or suggest another cause for the diplopia. For example, a lesion in the region of the trochlear nucleus in the midbrain might produce an ipsilateral Horner syndrome as well as a contralateral fourth nerve palsy. The presence of other cranial nerve palsies ipsilateral to a fourth nerve palsy suggests a cavernous sinus, superior orbital fissure, or orbital apex lesion. The presence of brainstem signs or intorsion of the hypertropic eye suggests a skew deviation rather than a fourth nerve palsy. The presence of areflexia or ataxia may suggest Miller-Fisher syndrome. The presence of fluctuating signs, such as ptosis, suggests myasthenia gravis, while the presence of exophthalmos or lid retraction suggests thyroid-associated (Graves') ophthalmopathy.

In our opinion, initial neuroimaging is not essential in patients with congenital fourth nerve palsy, isolated fourth nerve palsy due to head trauma, or isolated acute-onset fourth nerve palsy in association with vascular risk factors. We believe, however, that neuroimaging should be performed in all other patients and in those with a presumed microvascular etiology who do not recover within 3 months, although even then the imaging will rarely be abnormal if there are no other neurologic signs. In patients greater than 50 years old with a presumed microvascular etiology, you should ask about symptoms of giant cell arteritis and investigate urgently if any are present.

Treatment is directed toward the underlying cause. Although most patients with an isolated and presumed microvascular fourth nerve palsy will completely recover within 3 months, you should address their vascular risk factors and consider starting low-dose aspirin to reduce the risk of future vascular events. A Fresnel prism can minimize diplopia in patients who do not completely recover. Alternatively, patients with disabling diplopia that is both longstanding and stable could be offered surgery; inferior oblique myectomy or recession is often the most appropriate procedure in these cases.

Summary

* Head trauma, congenital deficit, and microvascular ischemic mononeuropathy are the most common causes of an isolated fourth nerve palsy.

* Familiarity with the Parks-Bielchowsky three-step test is essential in diagnosing a fourth nerve palsy.

* Most patients with an isolated and presumed microvascular fourth nerve palsy will completely recover within 3 months but underlying vascular risk factors should be evaluated and treated.

* A Fresnel prism can minimize diplopia in patients who do not completely recover. Alternatively, patients with disabling diplopia that is both longstanding and stable could be offered strabismus surgery.

Bibliography

Brazis PW. Palsies of the trochlear nerve: diagnosis and localization: recent concepts. *Mayo Clin Proc.* 1993;68:501-509.

Brodsky MC, Donahue SP, Vaphiades M, Brandt T. Skew deviation revisited. *Surv Ophthalmol.* 2006;51:105-128.

Leigh RJ, Zee DS. *The Neurology of Eye Movements.* 4th ed. New York: Oxford University Press; 2006.

von Noorden GK, Murray E, Wong SY. Superior oblique paralysis: review of 270 cases. *Arch Ophthalmol.* 1986; 104:1771-1776.

41

WHAT IS THE APPROPRIATE EVALUATION IN A PATIENT SUSPECTED OF HAVING A SIXTH NERVE PALSY?

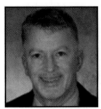

Steven R. Hamilton, MD

A 60-year-old man has binocular horizontal diplopia. He does not abduct OD well and has an incomitant esotropia. Now what?

The first step in evaluating a patient with diplopia is acquiring a solid and focused history. Your patient should describe binocular diplopia that is predominantly horizontal, present at distance more than at near, and typically worse looking to one side. There may only be diplopia looking to one side, such as while driving, and none with reading if the palsy is mild. Worrisome symptoms for intracranial disease such as tumor include intermittent or gradual onset particularly with progression, persistent pain over weeks, ipsilateral facial numbness or weakness, hearing changes, or vertigo.

One usually suspects a sixth nerve palsy based on the patient's history and the initial finding on examination of extraocular motility of an abduction deficit. Beware that all abduction deficits are not due to sixth nerve palsy and a number of other possibilities should be considered (Table 41-1). Those occurring most frequently are a restrictive ophthalmopathy due to thyroid eye disease or myopathy from myasthenia gravis.

You should look for orbital signs such as proptosis, chemosis, and lid edema during the exam. If abducting saccades are not obviously slow, one should perform forced ductions to rule out a restrictive process or consider orbital imaging with high-resolution computed tomography (CT) or magnetic resonance imaging (MRI). Myasthenia can mimic any cranial nerve palsy and you should consider a Tensilon test, particularly if there is any history or finding of ptosis of either or both eyes. In my experience, myasthenia rarely

---

Table 41-1
Etiology of Abduction Deficit

- Sixth nerve palsy
- Restrictive ophthalmopathy, such as thyroid eye disease
- Ocular myasthenia gravis
- Congenital: Duane's or Möbius syndrome
- Nonspecific orbital inflammation (pseudotumor)
- Entrapment of the medial rectus muscle from trauma
- Spasm of the near reflex

---

presents with an isolated abduction deficit; it more commonly affects adduction, mimicking an internuclear ophthalmoplegia or partial third nerve palsy. One could also obtain acetylcholine receptor antibody titers.

Once you determine the patient has a probable sixth nerve palsy, the work-up should proceed based on the patient's age, duration of symptoms, and the presence of any other worrisome symptoms as noted above or orbital, or other neurological signs. The latter would include looking for any other cranial nerve abnormalities or dysfunction of the oculosympathetic pathway (Horner syndrome). If other neurological signs are present, the patient should undergo contrast-enhanced cranial MRI. If there are any orbital signs such as proptosis, injection, chemosis, or a bruit, you should obtain an orbital and brain MRI with contrast, as well as magnetic resonance angiography (MRA) and magnetic resonance venography (MRV).

If the patient is 50 years or older, with sudden onset of symptoms, and no other orbital or neurological signs other than a sixth nerve palsy, and finally, has known vasculopathic risk factors such as diabetes, hypertension, or hyperlipidemia, you can presume an ischemic basis to the palsy. Regular follow-up checks at monthly intervals should be done documenting gradual resolution of the palsy. If any new signs or symptoms develop during this time or the palsy does not resolve within 3 months or progresses, a brain MRI with contrast must be performed. You should also consider screening any patient over 50 for the possibility of giant cell arteritis and obtain a Westergren erythrocyte sedimentation rate (ESR) and C-reactive protein.

Never forget that a patient is only allowed one ocular motor nerve palsy at a time on the basis of benign ischemia. Multiple cranial nerve palsies demand prompt neuroimaging with MRI with contrast with careful attention to the region of the superior orbital fissure and cavernous sinus.

I believe that patients under age 50 and those 50 or older without known vascular risk factors mandate careful neuroimaging with MRI of the brain with contrast, with orbital views, if there is any concern about an orbital process. This includes all sixth nerve palsies in young adults and children, since a high percentage of childhood sixth nerve palsies are secondary to compression from tumor (Table 41-2). MRA should be considered on occasion even with a normal brain MRI if aneurysm is suspected.

Table 41-2

Localization of Nonisolated Sixth Nerve Palsies

Sixth Palsy With the Following:	Localization	Examples
Ipsilateral gaze palsy +/- ipsilateral 7th palsy	6th nucleus in the pons	Stroke, glioma, multiple sclerosis
Ipsilateral 5th, 7th, Horner syndrome, or contralateral hemiparesis	6th nerve fascicle in pons	Stroke, tumor, multiple sclerosis
Ipsilateral deafness, vertigo, 5th or 7th palsy	Cerebellopontine (CP) angle	Tumors in CP angle
Ipsilateral otitis media and/or mastoiditis signs	Petrous apex	Mastoiditis
Ipsilateral 3rd, 4th, or 5th palsy or Horner syndrome	Cavernous sinus	Tumor, vascular fistula, thrombosis, infection, inflammation, aneurysm
Optic nerve dysfunction, +/- 3rd, 4th, or 5th cranial nerve dysfunction	Orbital apex	Tumor, infection, inflammation
Orbital signs (eg, proptosis)	Orbit	Tumor, infection, inflammation
Bilateral palsies	Nonlocalized	Often due to raised intracranial pressure or meningeal processes

Adapted from Pane A, Burdon M, Miller NR. *The Neuro-Ophthalmology Survival Guide.* New York, NY: Mosby; 2006:230-231.

A special case should be made for bilateral sixth nerve palsies, even if relatively asymmetric in degree. This finding should raise concern for increased intracranial pressure or meningeal disease (eg, inflammation, infection, neoplasm) and warrant immediate MRI with contrast and if negative, probably a diagnostic lumbar puncture with assessment of opening pressure and cerebrospinal fluid (CSF) profile.

Management of a transient sixth nerve palsy may include temporary patching of the eye or fogging a spectacle lens with semi-opaque tape. I have generally found that ischemic sixths do not really need a temporary prism given their short duration. For chronic sixths, prisms may be helpful, although ultimately strabismus surgery may be the best option. Surgery should not be considered until the palsy has been followed and remains stable for 6 to 12 months. I have had good success with surgery even for compressive etiologies such as cavernous sinus meningiomas that are inoperable. Botulinum toxin can be used as a temporizing measure, but as it dissipates, the diplopia will return.

Summary

* Sixth nerve palsy is but one cause of an abduction defct; be familiar with the differential diagnosis.

* Management of a transient (eg, ischemic) sixth nerve palsy may include temporary patching of the eye or fogging a spectacle lens with semi-opaque tape.

* Strabismus surgery may be the best option for patients with chronic deviations who fail or are intolerant of conservative measures.

Bibliography

Glaser JS. *Neuro-Ophthalmology*. 2nd ed. Philadelphia, PA: JB Lippincott Company; 1990:366.

Miller NR, Newman NJ, Biousse V, Kerrison JB. In: *Walsh and Hoyt's Clinical Neuro-Ophthalmology: The Essentials*. 2nd ed. New York, NY: JB Lippincott Co; 2008:404.

Pane A, Burdon M, Miller NR. *The Neuro-Ophthalmology Survival Guide*. New York, NY: Mosby; 2006:230-231.

42

How Do I Evaluate a Patient With Multiple Ocular Motor Cranial Nerve Palsies?

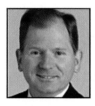

Greg Kosmorsky, DO

A 65-year-old man with diabetes complains of diplopia. He has what looks like a right partial third and sixth nerve palsy. What should I do now?

This particular patient presents a number of diagnostic challenges. One possibility is that the diplopia is due to microvascular ischemia. However, in general, ischemic cranial nerve palsies occur one at a time and resolve within 3 months. For instance, a diabetic patient can have a sixth nerve palsy that resolves, a third nerve palsy in the opposite side a few months later, and a peripheral seventh nerve palsy a number of months after that event. This clinical picture would be consistent with small vessel vasculopathy causing ischemic mononeuropathies. However, when you evaluate someone with multiple, ipsilateral, *simultaneous* ocular motor cranial nerve palsies, you must exclude an abnormality in the region of the cavernous sinus, superior orbital fissure, or perhaps within the orbit. Potential causes include vascular, neoplastic, infectious, and inflammatory disorders. However, to make things even more challenging, there are reports of multiple, ipsilateral simultaneous ocular motor cranial nerve palsies due to diabetes! Thus, the differential diagnosis is extensive (Table 42-1).

Approximately 50% of patients with a microvascular paresis experience significant pain/headache. The pain is centered in and about the eye and forehead, possibly with radiation to the vertex of the scalp or even to the occipital region. The pain is believed to arise from involvement of the trigeminal afferents that supply the meninges and blood vessels. Testing of the trigeminal nerve should be performed in each of its 3 divisions. In

Table 42-1

Causes of Acquired Multiple Ocular Motor Cranial Nerve Palsies and the Differential Diagnosis

1. Orbit

Idiopathic orbital inflammation (pseudotumor)
Contiguous sinusitis
Mucormycosis or other fungal infection
Metastatic tumor
Lymphoma/leukemia

2. Cavernous Sinus/Superior Orbital Fissure

Vascular
- Intracavernous carotid artery aneurysm
- Carotid-cavernous sinus fistula

Neoplasm
- Primary intracranial tumor
  - Pituitary adenoma
  - Meningioma
  - Craniopharyngioma
- Local metastases
  - Nasopharyngeal tumor
  - Squamous cell carcinoma
- Distant metastases
  - Lymphoma
  - Multiple myeloma
  - Carcinoma

Inflammation
- Bacterial
  - Sinusitis
  - Mucocele
  - Periostitis

- Viral
  - Herpes zoster
- Fungal
  - Mucormycosis
- Spirochetal
  - Treponema pallidum
- Mycobacterial
  - Mycobacterium tuberculosis
- Unknown cause:
  - Sarcoidosis
  - Wegener's granulomatosis
  - Tolosa-Hunt syndrome

3. Brain

Brainstem stroke
Carcinomatosis
Paraneoplastic effect

4. Miscellaneous

Fisher syndrome
Myasthenia gravis
Diabetic ophthalmoplegia
Giant cell arteritis
Thyroid eye disease

addition, examination should include evaluation of seventh nerve function. In the patient under discussion, I assume there is no facial weakness. However, if present, one should consider the possibility of an acquired myopathy such as myasthenia gravis or Fisher syndrome.

The patient's right optic nerve function also should be carefully assessed because of the possibility of an orbital apex syndrome, in which case the optic nerve as well as the ocular motor cranial nerves are affected. Careful evaluation of visual acuity, color vision, pupils, and visual fields must be performed, as well as examination of the optic discs. Any involvement of the optic nerve would therefore suggest that the lesion is located at the orbital apex and imaging would be directed to that specific area.

In the setting of multiple cranial neuropathies, neuroimaging is mandatory. Do not make your radiologist play "what am I thinking" but rather specify the topographic area of concern and the diagnostic possibilities. Contrast-enhanced magnetic resonance

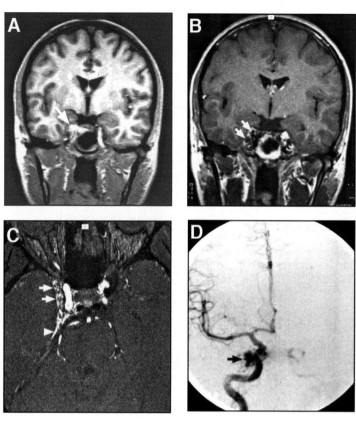

Figure 42-1. These MRIs and cerebral angiogram are that of an 18-year-old woman who presented with a painful right sixth nerve palsy. The MRIs were at first interpreted as normal. However, the clinical situation dictated a review of the images that demonstrated enlargement of the cavernous sinus on the right that on angiography proved to be a dural cavernous fistula. (A) Coronal T1 unenhanced image of the cavernous sinus reveals mild enlargement on the right (arrows). (B) Coronal T1 enhanced image of the cavernous sinus demonstrates multiple signal voids (arrows) within the cavernous sinus. (C) Axial MRA shows abnormal vasculature (arrows) within the right cavernous sinus. There is also increased signal along the dura of the tentorium cerebelli (arrowhead). (D) AP view of digital subtraction cerebral angiogram demonstrates fistula (arrow) within the right cavernous sinus.

imaging (MRI) is the procedure of choice. Generally, you want to get specific views of the orbit and cavernous sinus (Figure 42-1). I find coronal views to be particularly helpful, and fat-suppression techniques are essential in evaluating the orbit. Some institutions already have established protocols for specific cranial nerves, and if available, should be employed. Depending on the results of the MRI, other imaging techniques might be employed. For instance, if a large flow void is detected within the cavernous sinus, possibly due to an intracavernous carotid artery aneurysm, computed tomography angiography (CTA) or magnetic resonance angiography (MRA) should be performed. An enlarged superior ophthalmic vein may be due to a cavernous sinus fistula, in which case catheter angiography would be needed for both diagnosis and treatment.

When the radiologist deems the images to be "normal," other disease processes require consideration. Zoster ophthalmicus may affect multiple ocular motor cranial nerves with development of the typical skin rash. On occasion, however, zoster may present without a vesicular skin rash. Thyroid eye disease is also in the differential diagnosis with "normal" imaging as findings may be subtle or overlooked. On clinical examination one should look for evidence of proptosis, lid retraction and lag, engorgement of vessels over the extraocular muscles, and periorbital edema. Apical compression of the optic nerve is best appreciated on coronal gadolinium-enhanced views. A carotid dissection may occur spontaneously, creating ischemia in the cavernous sinus; however, such cases are very unusual. Dysguesia (an abnormal perception of taste) or pain in the neck/pretragal region could provide clues to a dissection. Myasthenia gravis can certainly present with unilateral ophthalmoplegia; ask and look for evidence of systemic weakness and consider obtaining acetylcholine receptor antibody titers and performing an intravenous Tensilon test. The most sensitive test for myasthenia is the single-fiber electromyogram, a test that is not widely available. The possibility of mucormycosis must be considered in diabetic and immunosuppressed patients. This process often affects diabetics with ketosis and an eschar may be seen in the nose. There is usually a rapid progression of clinical signs and it can cause death if left untreated. Invasion of the cavernous sinus by other fungi, especially *Aspergillus* species, may also occur.

Treatment will depend upon results of diagnostic studies. If our patient's ophthalmoplegia is due to diabetes, her imaging will be normal and her diplopia should resolve in 3 months. If it does not, the patient must be fully re-evaluated. That, being said, there are unusual cases of persistent cranial neuropathies from a small vessel vasculopathy. If repeated imaging and other studies are negative, consideration might be given for strabismus surgery.

Summary

* In the setting of multiple cranial neuropathies, neuroimaging is mandatory.

* Do not make your radiologist play "what am I thinking" but rather specify the topographic area of concern and the diagnostic possibilities.

* Contrast-enhanced cranial MRI is the initial diagnostic procedure of choice.

Bibliography

Eshaugh CG, Siatkowski RM, Smith JL, Kline LB. Simultaneous, multiple cranial neuropathies in diabetes mellitus. *J Neurooophtahlmol.* 1995;15(4):219-24

Johnston JL. Parasellar syndromes. *Curr Neurol Neurosci Rep.* 2002;2(5):423-31

Bennett JL, Pelak VS. Palsies of the third, fourth, and sixth cranial nerves. *Ophthalmol Clin North Am.* 2001;14(1): 169-85

Bianchi-Marzoli S, Brancato R. Third, fourth, and sixth cranial nerve palsies. *Curr Opin Ophthalmol.* 1997;8(6):45-51

Hamilton SR. Neuro-ophthalmology of eye movement disorders. *Curr Opin Ophthalmol.* 1999;10(6):405-10

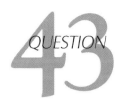

43

WHAT IS BLEPHAROSPASM?

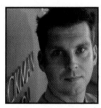

Timothy J. McCulley, MD
(co-authored with Thomas N. Hwang, MD, PhD)

*A 50-year-old woman complains of increasing bilateral blinking. It sometimes involves contrac-
tion of her face, too. What should be done? Does a scan need to be done?*

A muscle spasm is an abnormal, involuntary muscular contraction. Blepharospasm
refers to a spasm of the eyelid or, more specifically, the orbicularis oculi and brow depressors. There are many causes of blepharospasm, including more generalized dystonias,
hemifacial spasm, and ocular irritation, such as dry eye disease. When occurring primarily and in isolation, the term *benign essential blepharospasm* is applied.

The cause of benign essential blepharospasm is not clear. Most think blepharospasm is
a focal dystonia resulting from a disorder of the basal ganglia. However, substantial clinical evidence for brainstem dysfunction also exists. It has been suggested that brainstem
interneurons controlling eyelid closure may be hyperexcitable. Alternatively, the brainstem excitability might be facilitated by a primary basal ganglia disorder. More recently,
patients with blepharospasm have been assessed with functional imaging studies. Test
results have failed to uniformly implicate the basal ganglia and have located multiple
other areas of abnormal function within the brainstem as well as cortical area. This suggests the possibility that essential blepharospasm may be the common phenotype of a
number of contributing abnormalities.

Blepharospasm is usually gradual in onset and initially appears as excessive blinking. Most cases are bilateral from onset but occasionally may be asymmetric or initially
unilateral, with fellow eye involvement following shortly thereafter. Initially, it may be

minimally symptomatic and often first noticed by a spouse or family member. Rarely, more than one member of a family is affected.

Photophobia may be an accompanying symptom and in rare cases may precede noticeable spasms. Disease progression varies greatly. With some cases, it never advances beyond being a nuisance, whereas with others, it can become visually crippling. "Functional blindness" can occur in severe cases where patients become unable to open their eyes for hours at a time.

In most instances, no significant exacerbating or relieving factors are identifiable. Probably the most common exacerbating factor is light, and these patients may find some relief with filtered glasses. Stress, fatigue, and concentration may aggravate the disease in others. Conversely, rest and relaxation may help.

After a history for potentially causative factors is taken, your patient should be evaluated for secondary causes of blepharospasm like ocular irritation, dry eyes, or allergy. Medications that can be associated with dystonia should also be recorded. Common ones include those used to treat Parkinson's disease and most neuroleptics.

Initial evaluation in your patient should include a careful ocular examination for possible sources of ocular irritation. The assessment for dry eye disease includes slit lamp evaluation of the cornea and measurement of tear production. Misdirected lashes, blepharitis, and signs of allergic conjunctivitis should be noted. If any of the above signs are detected, the blepharospasm may be secondary to irritation. Such irritants may exacerbate the disease even in patients with essential blepharospasm.

I also recommend that patients should have a complete neurological history with attention paid particularly to the cranial nerve examination. Compressive lesions of the facial nerve and even less commonly brainstem neoplasm may result in spasms of the facial musculature, including the orbicularis oculi. In such cases, dysfunction of adjacent nerves can be encountered. In nonisolated cases associated with any neurological findings, further evaluation is warranted. Otherwise, I do not recommend imaging in patients with isolated benign essential blepharospasm.

Your patient complains of occasional spasms of her face in addition to the blepharospasm, raising the possibility of a more diffuse process, which may require imaging studies. The most commonly associated syndromes include Meige syndrome and hemifacial spasm. Meige syndrome (oromandibular dystonia) is a bilateral movement disorder that, in addition to blepharospasm, can involve the jaw muscles (jaw clenching or mouth opening), lips (grimacing), and tongue (protrusion). However, patients with blepharospasm can have variable degrees of facial and neck involvement, and the distinction between benign essential blepharospasm and Meige syndrome is not always clear. These disorders may prove to represent extremes of the same disease. Regardless, degenerative diseases and compressive lesions can present with movement disorders resembling Meige syndrome. In my opinion, therefore, imaging should be considered for patients with involvement of the lower face.

The distinguishing feature of hemifacial spasm is that it is invariably unilateral. Various muscles served by the facial nerve are involved. Spasms of the lower face (orbicularis ori) and neck (platysma) are common. I recommend an evaluation for a compressive lesion for these patients. A small aberrant artery often compresses the root of the facial nerve as it exits the brainstem.

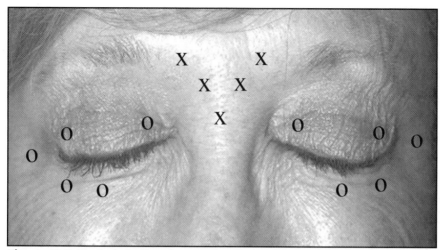

Figure 43-1. Typical starting dose and pattern of Botox injection for the treatment of blepharospasm. Each "X" marks the site of a single 4 unit injection. Each "O" marks the site of a 2 unit injection. Risk of blepharoptosis is reduced by avoiding the central upper eyelid. Also, there is a trend toward avoiding the medial lower eyelid, which carries increased risk of affecting the underlying inferior oblique muscle.

Any source of irritation is treated first when a secondary cause for blepharospasm is found. Consideration can also be given to tinted glasses. Although controversial, chromatic lenses (FL-41) designed specifically for the treatment of blepharospasm are commercially available.

Botulinum toxin injection (Botox, Allergan, Irvine, CA) is the mainstay of therapy for most patients. Numerous variations of dosage and injection location have been proposed. Figure 43-1 gives a typical regimen that is employed by the authors. However, the precise treatment strategy is tailored based on spasm location. For example, some may require treatment of the brow depressors (glabella) whereas others may not. Those with more muscle mass or stronger contractions may require higher doses. A typical starting dose would be 10 units per eye and, if needed, 20 units for the medial brow depressors. If insufficient, the dose is increased with subsequent treatments. The interval of treatment varies and should be tailored to individual patient needs. An adequate dose usually lasts roughly 3 months and in some up to 6 months or more. I recommend using the lowest effective dose and least frequent treatment interval to minimize the risk of developing resistance. Although less effective, botulinum type B (Myobloc [Solstice Neurosciences, Inc, San Francisco, CA]) can be tried in patients who develop resistance to Botox.

There have been inconsistent anecdotal reports of successful treatment with systemic medications. These are worth trying in patients resistant or opposed to treatment with Botox. More commonly used medications include gabapentin, diazepam, clonazepam, baclofen, carbamazepine, levodopa and carbidopa, and benztropine.

As a last resort, surgery may be considered. Orbicularis oculi myectomy is effective when correctly performed. However, it can be disfiguring and wrought with complications. Simple removal of excess eyelid skin (blepharoplasty) may allow the brow to be recru'' d for eyelid elevation. However, the effect of this is limited and probably inconsequential in most severe cases.

Summary

* Blepharospasm and hemifacial spasm are distinct clinical entities with characteristic clinical findings.
* Botulinum injections may provide relief for symptomatic patients.
* Surgical treatments are generally considered as a last resort.

Bibliography

Anderson RL, Patel BC, Holds JB, Jordan DR. Blepharospasm: past, present, and future. *Ophthal Plast Reconstr Surg.* 1998;14:305-317.

Baker RS, Andersen AH, Morecraft RJ, Smith CD. A functional magnetic resonance imaging study in patients with benign essential blepharospasm. *J Neuroophthalmol.* 2003;23:11-15.

Scott AB. Development of botulinum toxin therapy. *Dermatol Clin.* 2004;22:131-133.

44

WHAT IS HEMIFACIAL SPASM?

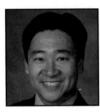

Michael S. Lee, MD
(co-authored with Andrew R. Harrison, MD)

The patient is a 40-year-old man who is reporting a 2-year history of episodic, involuntary closure of his left eye, and a 6-month history of contractions of the remainder of the left side of his face. His general health is excellent and he takes no medication regularly. With the exception of the involuntary movement of the left side of his face, his examination is normal. What evaluation is necessary?

We think that your patient might have hemifacial spasm (HFS). HFS manifests as involuntary, episodic contractions of the muscles innervated by the facial nerve. Almost always unilateral, the peak presentation occurs between the ages of 40 to 60 years and more commonly affects women. It often begins with isolated orbicularis oculi involvement and over months to years gradually spreads to the rest of the ipsilateral facial muscles. The spasms tend to be synchronous (ie, all of the muscles contract simultaneously). Spasms increase in frequency with stress, fatigue, anxiety, and voluntary facial contractions. You can often bring out the spasms by having the patient forcefully close his or her eyes for several seconds. One of the distinguishing features from other involuntary facial movements is that the spasms continue during sleep.

The most common cause of HFS is compression of the facial nerve as it exits the brainstem by an anomalous or aberrant vessel (Figure 44-1). While patients with HFS initially appear normal between contractions, it is not unusual for these patients to develop mild to moderate facial weakness with long-standing HFS because of the compression of the seventh nerve. Other less common (<1%) causes include posterior fossa tumors such as an epidermoid, meningioma, or brainstem glioma.

Figure 44-1. Axial MRA source image demonstrates vascular compression (V) of the seventh nerve (7th) as it exits the pons (P).

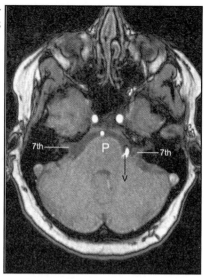

Other involuntary facial movements should be considered when making the diagnosis of HFS. Unilateral twitching of the facial muscles may occur following a seventh nerve palsy secondary to aberrant regeneration of the peripheral nerve fibers with synkinesis. The patient will have a history of Bell's palsy and if you look closely, the contractions tend to be asynchronous. For example, the eye closure may occur moments before the corner of the mouth or vice versa. Eyelid myokymia appears as involuntary undulating movements of one eyelid at a time. The eye does not close and the twitches last only seconds. The direction of the twitches may be horizontal. Tics generally involve males in their second decade of life. These are not typically isolated to unilateral facial contraction. There may be intermittent eye deviation, shrugging, or throat clearing. These do not persist during sleep and they often resolve spontaneously by age 20 years. Blepharospasm involves both eyes and may appear as excessive blinking or forceful eyelid closure. Finally, neuroleptic agents may also result in unusual facial movements. These movements are generally bilateral and asynchronous. We would recommend that you look in the patient's mouth since the tongue is often involved (this does not occur in typical HFS).

Your patient's age and clinical history are consistent with hemifacial spasm. The cause of his HFS is overwhelmingly in favor of irritation of the seventh nerve by an aberrant vessel. Although neuroimaging is low yield, there are several well-documented cases of HFS from tumors. We believe that magnetic resonance imaging (MRI) and magnetic resonance angiography (MRA) with attention to the cerebellopontine angle and facial nerve should be performed. These scans will allow us to rule out posterior fossa tumors and if present, may demonstrate vascular compression of the pons or facial nerve.

We generally treat patients with debilitating HFS with subcutaneous injections of botulinum toxin type A (Figure 44-2). We usually start with 2.5 units per injection. Preinjection topical anesthetic or an ice pack may reduce pain. We try to avoid the area around and below the nasolabial fold because of the risk of orbicularis oris weakness. Many patients prefer injections around the eye alone for this reason. Patients should understand that the risk of double vision and ptosis may occur in 2% to 8%. For this reason, they should avoid rubbing the injection areas or lying down for the first several hours after they leave the

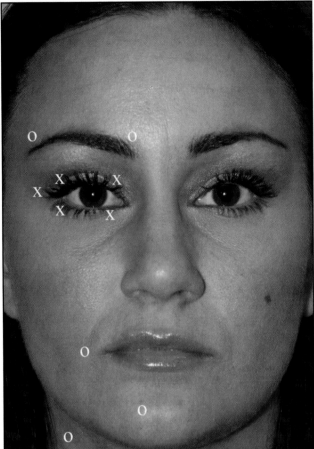

Figure 44-2. Injection sites for botulinum toxin A in a patient with HFS. The injection dose is typically 2.5 to 5 units. Typical (X) and optional (O) injection sites are shown depending on the individual findings and desires.

office to avoid unwanted spread of the botulinum toxin. Bruising is common and often inevitable. For the first few weeks, we encourage aggressive lubrication with artificial tears and ointment at bedtime for exposure keratopathy secondary to lagophthalmos. Improvement in spasms occurs in approximately 3 to 7 days and typically persists for 3 to 6 months after which the patient must return for repeat injections. We do not favor oral medications such as benzodiazepines (eg, clonazepam), anticonvulsants (eg, carbamazepine), or muscle relaxants (eg, baclofen). We have found that these are not that effective and result in undesirable side effects.

We also inform patients that neurosurgical intervention is another consideration. Via suboccipital craniectomy, a Teflon sponge can be placed between the compressive vessel and the seventh nerve. This has a high rate of success (up to 90%) and is curative in many cases, but carries a risk of facial palsy, ipsilateral deafness, vertigo, and stroke. Recurrences of HFS after surgery have been reported in up to 20%. In our experience, most patients prefer botulinum toxin injections.

Summary

* Hemifacial spasm is a clinical diagnosis.

* Magnetic resonance imaging might be useful to exclude a compressive lesion.

* Botulinum toxin injections are useful in symptomatic patients.

* Neurosurgical intervention is another therapeutic consideration but has significant risks.

Bibliography

Costa J, Espirito-Santo C, Borges A, et al. Botulinum toxin type A therapy for hemifacial spasm. *Cochrane Database Syst Rev.* 2005;25:CD004899.

Samii M, Gunther T, Iaconetta G, et al. Microvascular decompression to treat hemifacial spasm: long term results for a consecutive series of 143 patients. *Neurosurgery.* 2002;50:712-718.

Tan NC, Chan LL, Tan EK. Hemifacial spasm and involuntary facial movements. *Q J Med.* 2002;95:493-500.

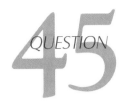

HOW DO YOU DEAL WITH NONORGANIC VISUAL LOSS?

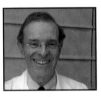

Robert L. Lesser, MD

A 13-year-old girl reports that her vision is "just not clear." She noted this problem at the beginning of the school year and has trouble "reading for a long time." The exam shows that her visual acuity is 20/50 in the right eye and 20/20 in the left eye with an inferior visual field defect in the right eye (Figure 45-1). The remainder of her exam is normal with no afferent pupillary defect; the optic nerves and maculae look healthy. Another eye care provider has prescribed reading glasses, but these were of little help. What are the next steps in evaluating this patient?

When I am dealing with unexplained visual loss, normally I recommend considering the subtle but recognizable causes for unexplained visual loss. I have listed the major considerations in Table 45-1.

If no abnormality is found on the clinical examination, then the possibility of a nonorganic cause becomes more likely.

You should develop a specific "game plan" in approaching a patient with a potentially nonorganic basis for diminished vision. I would recommend that you develop a sympathetic, but direct approach in proving that visual function is normal. Numerous testing techniques have been proposed in dealing with this clinical problem. It is essential that you select a series of these techniques and become facile in performing them. Showmanship might even be required, but above all, reassurance and encouragement of the patient are keys to success.

My favorite tests to detect nonorganic vision loss from the simplest to most complex include the following.

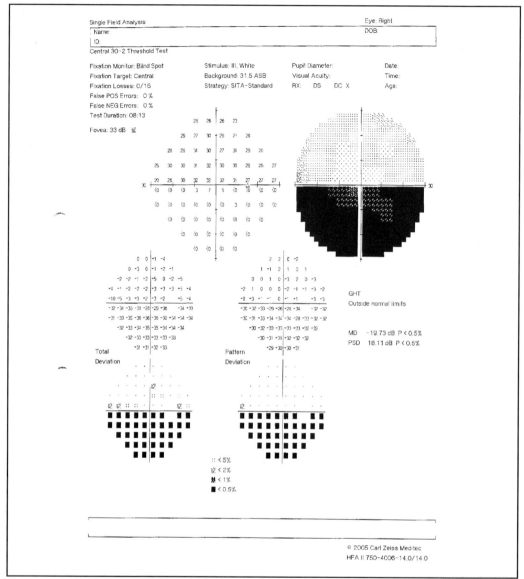

Figure 45-1. Automated visual field demonstrates inferior visual field loss in the right eye.

Stereo Acuity Testing

If you document 40 seconds of arc, then the patient has 20/20 vision. Sixty seconds of arc is equivalent to 20/40, while 40 seconds indicates 20/20 acuity.

Near Distance Disparity

Look for a disparity in near and distance vision. If a patient can read 20/20 at near and 20/50 at distance, then the visual loss is not physiologic.

Table 45-1

Subtle or Easily Missed Causes for Unexplained Visual Loss

Cornea

  1. Irregular astigmatism
  2. Keratoconus
  3. Anterior basement membrane dystrophy

Lens

  1. Subtle cataracts—oil droplet, minimal nuclear sclerosis

Retina

  1. Occult macular dystrophy
  2. Cone dystrophy
  3. Paraneoplastic retinopathy
  4. Early Stargardt's disease
  5. Occult epiretinal membrane, macular hole, or edema

Optic Nerve

  1. Toxic or nutritional optic neuropathy
  2. Autosomal dominant optic atrophy

Prism Dissociation Test

Two alternate techniques are useful. The first involves placing a 4-diopter prism base-down in front of the "bad eye" and a 0.5 prism diopter base-down in front of the "good eye." The patient is then asked if he or she sees 2 lines. In this case, the patient will be shown the 20/20 line and asked to read each of them. He or she can read the top line forwards and the bottom line backwards. If your patient can do that, you have demonstrated he or she can see 20/20 from the "bad eye" (Figure 45-2A).

This is one of my favorite tests because it can be done quickly. Patients are usually fooled by this test because they are complaining of visual loss not diplopia.

An alternate method is to place a 4 prism diopter prism base-down in front of the better eye with both eyes open. The patient again is asked what he or she sees on the Snellen chart. If 2 lines of letters are seen and both lines are read correctly, then the patient has 20/20 vision in both eyes. Should the patient see only one line, then he or she may indeed have an organic basis for diminished vision in one eye (Figure 45-2B).

Regardless of the technique, this test must be carried out in an efficient and encouraging manner.

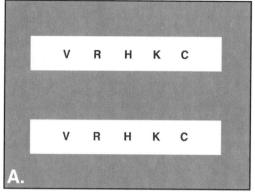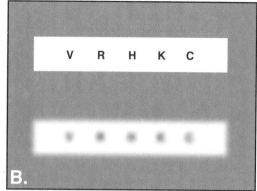

Figure 45-2. Prism dissociation test. (A) With good vision in each eye, the patient will be able to read each 20/20 line. (B) With poor vision in one eye, only one clear image of the 20/20 line will be seen. Often a second blurred image will be seen depending on the level of vision in the eye with an organic cause for reduced acuity.

Microscopic Killer Refraction (Toothpaste Refraction—Squeeze It Out Of Them)

Start at the 20/10 level for refraction and work up slowly using various "aids" such as red-green colors on the chart, rotating prism, Jackson cross cylinder, and lenses with minimal power (eg, ±0.25 or ±0.50). Then work up and go to the 20/15 line and repeat the same process. Use various aids to suggest that they will help, like pinhole, Risley prism, and "telescopic" lens.

You often need to take your time so you can wear the patient down; be creative and persuasive. By the time you get to the 20/20 level, the patient is instructed to read the "large letters." Show the patient multiple 20/20 lines and ask him or her to read the top line only. Using these techniques, with a little encouragement and positive reinforcement, a patient will often be able to read the 20/20 line.

Asymmetrical Fogging

Blur both eyes with the phoropter and then gradually dial lenses back to the correct refraction in front of the "bad eye" while keeping the good eye blurred. When patients read 20/20 from the "bad eye," you have made the diagnosis. The problem with this test is that patients will often close one eye figuring out how to beat the test. You can also use Polaroid lenses or red-green filters to dissociate the 2 eyes.

Different Distances

Measure acuity at different distances. If the patient can see 20/10 at 10 feet, that is equivalent to seeing 20/20 at 20 feet.

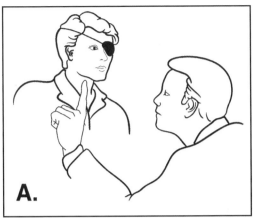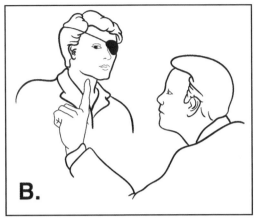

Figure 45-3. (A) Confrontation visual field testing with patient reporting inability to see fingers in inferior visual field. (B) Patient looking in direction of inferior visual field when told saccades are being tested, confirming that the patient indeed can see in the inferior visual field.

Saccade Envy Visual Field Test

The saccade envy test is a good way to prove that your patient's field loss is not real. First, perform confrontation visual field testing (Figure 45-3A). Next ask her to look at your finger in the periphery and then back at your nose. Tell her that these are some of the fastest saccades that you have ever seen! Praise these fast eye movements and bring some office personnel or other physicians in to observe and admire these unusually fast saccades. When demonstrating these "amazing" saccades, hold your finger in different "nonseeing areas" (Figure 45-3B). If the patient can see your fingers in these areas when testing saccades, then you have documented that her visual field loss is on a nonorganic basis.

Electrophysiologic Testing

If the above examination techniques are inconclusive, then electrophysiologic studies, such as electroretinogram (ERG) and visual evoked potential (VEP), are helpful.

It is essential to monitor visual fixation during these tests since you can get a false-positive result if the patient does not look at the stimulus correctly. If full-field ERG and pattern-reversal VEP are normal, then it is likely that the patient has nonorganic visual loss. At times, multifocal ERG testing may also be required to exclude a localized macular disorder.

Always remember that nonorganic visual loss is a diagnosis of exclusion. The patient may have an organic cause for diminished visual acuity that may be subtle and challenging to demonstrate. Further, the patient may have a superimposed "functional overlay," magnifying and embellishing the true deficit. You must tease apart the organic from the nonorganic! You must be certain not to overlook the cause of the patient's visual complaint; if there is any doubt, 1 or 2 follow-up visits may be advisable to confirm the diagnosis.

Most patients can be treated with reassurance often during the initial as well as 1 to 2 follow-up visits. A confrontational approach is usually counterproductive. It is essential to provide the patient with a "way out." Although psychiatric referral is usually not needed, physicians should be aware of the possibility of physical or sexual abuse associated with this condition in children. You should alert the pediatrician about the diagnosis.

Summary

* Most patients with nonorganic visual loss can be treated with reassurance often during the initial as well as 1 to 2 follow-up visits.
* A confrontational approach is usually counterproductive.
* Provide the patient with a "way out."
* Be aware of the possibility of physical or sexual abuse associated with this condition in children.

Bibliography

Bain KE, Beatty S, Lloyd C. Nonorganic visual loss in children. *Eye.* 2000;14:770-772.

Bengtzen R, Woodward M, Lynn MJ, Newman NJ, Biousse V. The "sunglasses sign" predicts nonorganic visual loss in neuro-ophthalmologic practice. *Neurology.* 2008;70:218-221.

Golnik KC, Lee AG, Eggenberger ER. The monocular vertical prism dissociation test. *Am J Ophthalmol.* 2004;137: 135-137.

Lim SA, Siatkowski RM, Farris BK. Functional visual loss in adults and children patient characteristics, management, and outcomes. *Ophthalmology.* 2005;112:1821-1828.

Trobe JD. *The Neurology of Vision.* New York, NY: Oxford University Press; 2001:369-388.

HOW DO YOU DIAGNOSE AND MANAGE MIGRAINE AURA?

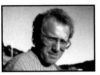

Robert H. Spector, MD

The patient has what sounds like the visual aura of migraine. She sees a jagged line in her peripheral vision that gets bigger over about 5 minutes and then moves across her visual field. However, she denies headache and has no previous history of migraine headaches. Can this still be migraine?

Aura is defined as a sensory warning that usually announces the onset of a more explicit neurological event, like a migraine headache or a major motor seizure. Visual auras in migraine may manifest as a transient negative scotoma (eg, homonymous hemianopia), monocular visual loss, or as a positive scotoma (eg, a luminous, colorful display of sparkling, dazzling, dancing, or flickering lights arrayed geometrically in homonymous portions of the visual field). While most migrainous auras herald the onset of a headache, 13% of migraineurs have the visual symptoms without headache, in which case the isolated visual experience is nosologically referred to as migraine aura without headache (acephalgic migraine).

An isolated, transient homonymous hemianopia, visual illusion, or visual hallucination can be caused by other conditions besides migraine. Thus, it behooves you to know the characteristic features of a migrainous aura and to know when and how aggressively to pursue other etiologies, when sufficient doubt exists.

The prototypic migraine aura begins as a small flickering ill-defined spot eccentric to fixation. The patient may be aware of something obscuring vision but often has difficulty describing it. Over 15 to 30 minutes, the obscuration enlarges and marches across the homonymous portions of visual field, leaving behind a wake of blindness that slowly fills in as the scintillation fades into the temporal periphery of the ipsilateral eye. If your patient claims that his or her experience was monocular, ask him or her to cover each eye independently at the onset of the next attack because he or she will often see a nasal defect or display in the less involved eye, thus establishing the symptoms as homonymous and more likely due to migraine.

Additional subtleties of the history that help to confirm the diagnosis of migraine aura without headache include the following: if the aura was preceded by or followed by another type of migraine accompaniment, such as paresthesias (pins and needles) that marched up one extremity and crossed to the other side; if certain situations predictably provoke visual symptoms or headache, like sleeplessness, hunger, alcohol consumption, or menses; a history of previous migraine headaches, with or without aura, as the syndrome of migraine aura without headache often occurs in patients who have had other types of migraine; and whether 2 or more identical episodes have occurred, especially months or years apart, with full recovery each time.

In contrast to the characteristic features of a migraine aura, the following atypical historical points or physical findings should alert you to the possibility of an alternative etiology: visual symptoms exclusively confined to the same side of the visual field; visual aura accompanied by a change in consciousness or followed by a persistent visual deficit, hemiparesis, hemisensory loss, or incontinence; monocular or bitemporal visual symptoms; or a recent flurry of transient symptoms with different neuro-ophthalmological manifestations (eg, an homonymous hemianopia one time and a transient hemiparesis or hemisensory loss another time).

Virtually all patients with transient visual phenomena see a physician after their vision has returned to normal. Accurate diagnosis, therefore, is predicated on meticulous history taking and the following observations during your physical examination: auscultation of the orbits, cranial vault, and neck vessels to listen for a bruit; direct and indirect ophthalmoscopy of both eyes to look for intravascular plugs or plaques, isolated or multiple retinal infarctions, or signs of venous stasis retinopathy; and quantitative visual field testing to detect an asymptomatic defect that topographically localizes to the retrochiasmal visual pathways.

An atypical history or the foregoing physical findings warrant a thorough evaluation of the following conditions: focal epilepsy, recurrent microemboli, structural lesions of the occipital lobe (arteriovenous malformation or brain tumor), hematological disorders, and collagen vascular disease. I also have a lower threshold for pursuing the differential diagnosis in the elderly because they often cannot recount the small, but characteristic details of their visual experience, and thromboembolism is more prevalent in their age group. That said, if the description of a transient visual event is sufficiently characteristic of migraine (build-up, march, and duration), I have yet to find an alternative etiology, which has over years of experience led me to the conclusion that very few nonmigrainous conditions mimic a characteristic migraine aura without headache.

Differentiating migraine from focal epilepsy may sometimes be difficult, particularly in children, since each condition may cause paroxysmal symptoms that march over time. Frequently, however, occipital epileptogenic discharges also produce tonic deviation of the eyes, vomiting, and a unilateral or generalized convulsion. Thromboembolism may indeed cause a transient homonymous hemianopia and should be considered in the elderly or in persons with evidence of arteriosclerotic risk factors (smoking, obesity, diabetes, hypertension, dyslipidemia, family predilection for premature vascular disease) or cardiac conditions that may cause thromboembolism (eg, valvular damage, recent myocardial infarction, cardiomyopathy). I was taught the clinical adage that vertebrobasilar artery disease commonly causes transient homonymous hemianopia and blindness, yet it occurs as the isolated manifestation in less than 2% of cases.

Although build-up, march, and duration help to distinguish a migraine aura, 25% of migraineurs state that their visual loss or display becomes maximum immediately. The absence of build-up should not exclude migraine but should at least engender a consideration of the differential diagnosis. In a thromboembolic transient ischemic attack (TIA), the sensory loss on the face, arm, and leg occur simultaneously, while the march of sensory symptoms in migraine gradually spreads over the face, fingers, or hand and migrates and crosses to the contralateral face and hand over 30 minutes. In general, the duration of a migrainous aura lasts 15 to 25 minutes, whereas 95% of TIAs last less than 15 minutes.

In my opinion, the indications for doing a magnetic resonance imaging (MRI) scan of the brain with and without contrast administration and/or MR angiography (MRA) of the intracranial or extracranial vessels in persons with migraine aura without headache or other headache syndromes include the following: atypical history or physical findings, rapidly increasing frequency and/or severity of auras alone or headaches, first or "worst" headache ever experienced, thunderclap or abrupt-onset incapacitating headache, new onset of headache or migraine aura without headache after age 50, and a headache or headaches that are refractory to traditional treatment.

Differential diagnosis of transient physical phenomena in the presence of normal imaging studies includes thrombocythemia, thrombotic thrombocytopenia, polycythemia, and other hyperviscosity states or clotting disorders.

Once confident that you are dealing with the diagnosis of migraine aura without headache, the treatments of choice are reassurance, reassurance, and more reassurance. Sometimes telling the patient to rebreathe their own air abbreviates or aborts the visual symptoms because increased blood carbon dioxide levels cause cerebral vasodilation, and theoretically should reverse the visual pathway dysfunction possibly caused by migrainous cerebral vasoconstriction. If visual symptoms become so frequent as to interfere with the quality of life of the patient, referral to a neurologist for further treatment is warranted.

Summary

* Migraine aura is a clinical diagnosis.
* Once confident that you are dealing with the correct diagnosis of migraine aura without headache, the treatment of choice is reassurance, reassurance, and more reassurance.
* If visual symptoms become so frequent as to interfere with the quality of life of the patient, referral to a neurologist should be considered.

Bibliography

Evans RW, Rozen TD, Adelman JU. Neuroimaging and other diagnostic testing in headache. In: Silberstein SD, Lipton RB, Delassio DJ, eds. *Wolff's Headaches and Other Pain.* 7th ed. New York, NY: Oxford University Press; 2001:27-49.

Fisher CM. Late-life migraine accompaniments as a cause of unexplained transient ischemic attacks. *Can J Neurol Sci.* 1980;7:9-17.

Hupp SL, Kline LB, Corbett, JJ. Visual disturbances of migraine. *Surv Ophthalmol.* 1989;33:221-236.

Savitz SI, Caplan LR. Vetebrobasilar disease. *N Engl J Med.* 2005;352:2618-2626.

Spector RH. Migraine. Focal points. *Am Acad Ophthalmol.* 2000;28:1-12.

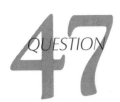

QUESTION 47

HOW DO I MANAGE THE LOW-FLOW CAROTID CAVERNOUS FISTULA?

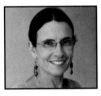

Leah Levi, MBBS

The patient is a 65-year-old elderly hypertensive woman with a chronic red eye. Topical anti-histamines, antibiotics, antivirals, and prednisone have been tried, but the eye just stays red. The vessels seem engorged, dilated, and tortuous. Now she is complaining of double vision and a "bulging" eye? What should be done?

In your patient, the engorged vessels, complaints of eye bulging, and diplopia tell you that this is not simple conjunctivitis. You should consider low-flow dural cavernous sinus fistula, which is a communication between one or more dural branches of the carotid artery and the cavernous sinus. As in your patient, this is generally painless with mild findings that at first can easily be mistaken for conjunctivitis or other common causes of red eye (Figure 47-1). Unlike high-flow fistulas, the patient often does not have a pulsatile or audible bruit.

Since the venous drainage of the eye and the orbit is impaired and under arterial pressure, you should systematically look for signs that reflect this increased venous pressure in 3 areas: 1) the eye itself, 2) the orbit, and 3) the cavernous sinus.

Eye

* Tortuous dilated conjunctival and episcleral vessels (Figure 47-2)
* Lid swelling and conjunctival chemosis
* Asymmetric intraocular pressure (higher on affected side)

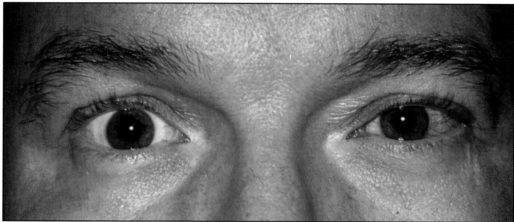

Figure 47-1. Mild red left eye in a patient with a low-flow dural fistula. In this case there was also a left Horner syndrome.

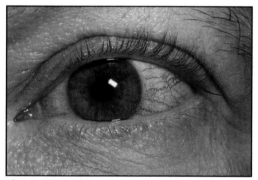

Figure 47-2. Dilated and tortuous conjunctival and episcleral veins in the patient from Figure 47-1. This patient's fistula closed spontaneously after a plane flight.

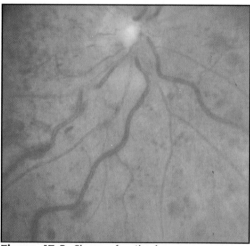

Figure 47-3. Signs of retinal venous congestion: dilated tortuous veins and hemorrhages. In this case there is also some mild disc edema.

* Increased pulse of applanation mires on affected side
* Retinal venous congestion (Figure 47-3)

The most common signs of a low-flow dural cavernous sinus fistula are found during ophthalmologic examination. In the eye the main effects of the increased venous pressure are the tortuosity of the conjunctival and episcleral vessels. There may even be some mild lid swelling and conjunctival chemosis. The increased episcleral venous pressure in turn leads to increased intraocular pressure compared to the unaffected eye, even to the abnormal range. A very useful sign I look for is increased pulsation of the Goldmann applanation mires on the affected side. Since the episcleral veins are under arterial pressure, there is a larger change in intraocular pressure from systole to diastole (increased pulse pressure). This sign helps me differentiate a fistula from other conditions that may have congestion as part of the clinical picture such as thyroid-associated orbitopathy or

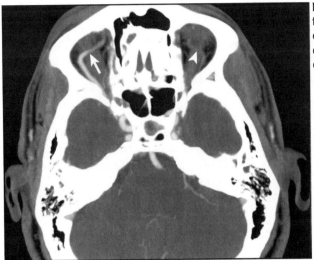

Figure 47-4. Dilated superior ophthalmic vein (arrow) in a right dural cavernous fistula. Note the normal diameter of the contralateral superior ophthalmic vein (arrowhead).

orbital inflammation. I also look for increased congestion and tortuosity of the retinal veins.

Orbit

∗ Proptosis (frequently absent or mild)

∗ Congestion of extraocular muscles (uncommon)

In the orbit, the increased venous pressure may cause proptosis on the affected side from orbital congestion. The extraocular muscles may be engorged in some cases and this can lead to diplopia.

Cavernous Sinus

∗ Ocular motor cranial nerve palsies (sixth the most common)

∗ Horner syndrome

Your patient's complaint of diplopia is from the effects of the increased venous pressure in the cavernous sinus, where the sixth nerve is commonly affected. In low-flow fistulas, the third nerve and fourth nerve may be involved but this is less common. Other possible signs to look for are an ipsilateral Horner syndrome (see Figure 47-1).

If the clinical findings suggest a low-flow dural cavernous sinus fistula, I usually obtain orbital imaging with contrast to confirm dilation of the superior ophthalmic vein (Figure 47-4). If you decide to obtain a magnetic resonance imaging (MRI) scan, make sure you ask for fat-saturated views of the orbits so that you can see the details of the superior ophthalmic vein. When ordering the imaging, I like to specify on the request that I suspect a fistula and to look for a dilated superior ophthalmic vein. MR angiography and computed tomography (CT) angiography can also be ordered to diagnose and better define the fistula. The choice of which modality to use is somewhat institution dependent, so it is worth speaking to the neuroradiologist regarding this.

Catheter angiography is still the definitive test for demonstrating the exact anatomy of the fistula. However, since up to 50% of low-flow dural fistulas close spontaneously and without complications within several months, and since angiography carries a small but definite risk, I usually do not obtain angiography when I first see the patient. This can always be done by the interventional neuroradiologist if the patient is referred for treatment.

Considering the high rate of spontaneous closure of the low-flow dural cavernous fistula, you can usually manage the patient conservatively, as long as the symptoms and findings are mild and not progressive or a danger to vision. If your patient has no concerning signs such as retinal venous congestion and has an intraocular pressure that can be controlled medically and is causing no visual field defects, then you can simply follow the patient, obtaining baseline visual field testing and fundus photography. I like to see the patient every few weeks to check the intraocular pressure, repeat the visual field testing, and make sure there are no signs of increasing retinal venous congestion. If your patient has proptosis and corneal exposure, I recommend lubricating drops and ointment. If your patient has diplopia, you can temporize with patching, Fresnel prism, or orthoptics depending on the clinical situation.

If the patient develops progressive and concerning signs such as increasing venous congestion, or intraocular pressure that is unable to be controlled medically or is causing visual field defects, or if the fistula does not close within a few months and the patient is symptomatic due to orbital congestion or diplopia, then I will refer to an interventional neuroradiologist for definitive treatment. Treatment consists of closing the communication between the arterial and venous systems. Depending on the exact anatomy this can be done either by introducing embolic materials into the arterial branches feeding the fistula or via the veins draining the fistula. In appropriate cases, coils or detachable balloons may be introduced via the superior ophthalmic vein by the interventional neuroradiologist coordinating with an orbital surgeon.

After closure of the fistula, whether spontaneously or after treatment, I like to document that the clinical findings have improved or resolved (as is usually the case), and manage any mild residual problems. Since occasionally the closure may not be complete or there may be a recurrence, I like to continue to follow these patients periodically, being prepared to manage mild findings or refer again to interventional neuroradiology for additional treatment.

Summary

* Patients with proptosis, ophthalmoplegia, and signs of orbital venous congestion should be evaluated for carotid cavernous sinus fistula.

* Consider referral of symptomatic patients to an interventional neuroradiologist for definitive evaluation and possible treatment.

* Closure of the communication between the arterial and venous systems can be done by endovascular techniques.

Bibliography

Liu HM, Wang YH, Chen YF, Cheng JS, Yip PK, Tu YK. Long-term clinical outcome of spontaneous carotid cavernous sinus fistulae supplied by dural branches of the internal carotid artery. *Neuroradiology.* 2001;43:1007-1014.

Miller NR. Diagnosis and management of dural carotid-cavernous sinus fistulas. *Neurosurg Focus.* 2007;23:E13.

HOW DO I RECOGNIZE LEBER'S HEREDITARY OPTIC NEUROPATHY?

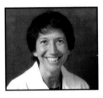

Nancy J. Newman, MD

The patient is a 22-year-old male in college who went out drinking over the weekend with his buddies and on Monday had loss of vision in the right eye to counting fingers vision. He had a right afferent pupillary defect and the nerve looked swollen on the right. A visual field was performed and showed a dense central scotoma on the right and was normal on the left. Optic neuritis was initially suspected and he was scheduled for magnetic resonance imaging (MRI) later in the week but now he is calling saying that he has vision loss in his left eye. Interestingly, the same thing happened to his brother last year at age 25 and his vision never really recovered. Any ideas?

This young man has suffered severe central visual loss in the right eye. The right relative afferent pupillary defect, the dense central scotoma, and the abnormal-appearing right optic nerve all led you to the appropriate localization of the problem to the right optic nerve. It was most certainly reasonable in a person of this age with an acute unilateral optic neuropathy to consider the possibility of inflammation of the optic nerve (ie, optic neuritis). However, if there was no pain at the time of visual loss, optic neuritis would be much less likely (over 90% of patients with optic neuritis will experience pain, usually on eye movement). Similarly, since optic neuritis tends to affect females far more often than males, I am always a bit wary of making a definitive diagnosis of typical idiopathic demyelinating optic neuritis in a man, especially when there is no complaint of pain. The real spoiler in this case is the loss of vision in the other eye within the week. Although optic neuritis can present in both eyes (and, indeed, the Optic Neuritis Treatment Trial showed that concurrent involvement in the fellow eye was not at all unusual, occurring in more than 40% of patients), the involvement of the second eye broadens the differential diagnosis to include infectious and other inflammatory etiologies of optic neuritis, such as syphilis and sarcoidosis, as well as other disease categories, including rapidly infiltrating neoplasms, such as the leukemias, lymphomas and malignant optic nerve gliomas, compressive lesions with rapid expansion such as pituitary apoplexy, or even vascular etiologies. However, the clinical presentation is most suggestive of Leber's hereditary optic neuropathy (LHON), and the history of a brother who suffered similar visual loss at age 25 essentially clinches the diagnosis.

LHON is a maternally inherited disorder, usually affecting individuals between the ages of 15 and 35 years, with a male predominance of 4 to 1. Onset is typically painless and acute or subacute, with simultaneous onset in both eyes in about 50% of cases, or sequential with an interval of days, weeks, or months. Essentially all patients have bilateral involvement by 1 year, typically by 6 months. Deterioration of vision in each eye has usually reached its nadir by 3 to 4 months, with most patients having visual acuities worse than 20/200. Visual field defects, as in this patient, are usually central or cecocentral scotomas. The classic funduscopic appearance in some LHON patients seen acutely is that of "pseudoedema" of the optic nerve head, in which the disc looks elevated, hyperemic, and swollen, but there is no late leakage on fluorescein angiography to indicate true disc edema. Small telangiectatic vessels may be seen on the disc and other retinal vessels may appear tortuous. These funduscopic changes may be seen not only in affected patients, but in "presymptomatic" individuals, and even in asymptomatic maternal relatives who never lose vision. However, many patients with LHON never manifest these funduscopic features, even when examined at the time of acute visual loss, occasionally resulting in an erroneous diagnosis of nonorganic visual loss in these patients. Ultimately, after several weeks, pallor of the optic nerve head and loss of nerve fiber layer supervenes. Magnetic resonance imaging is usually normal.

Typically, visual loss from LHON is permanent, although spontaneous recovery of even excellent central visual acuity can occur, especially in those patients who suffer their initial visual loss at a young age, usually less than 20 years, and who harbor one of the less common mitochondrial DNA mutations (see below). Visual recovery does not usually occur for at least 6 months to a year after visual loss, and often years later. Optic neuropathy is typically the only manifestation of the disease, although there are individuals and pedigrees with cardiac conduction defects and minor neurologic abnormalities.

LHON is inherited maternally; all offspring of a woman carrying the trait will inherit the trait, but only the females can pass the trait on to the subsequent generation. Maternal inheritance results when the genetic defect is in DNA that resides in the cytoplasm of the cell, rather than the nucleus, hence it is passed on via the mother's egg. This DNA resides in the mitochondria of the cell and is called mitochondrial DNA. Three point mutations in the mtDNA are considered to be causal in 90% to 95% of all cases of LHON and are designated "primary LHON mutations": the mutation at position 11778 within the mtDNA accounts for about 70% of LHON cases, the mutation at 3460 accounts for about 13% of LHON cases, and the mutation at 14484 accounts for about 14% of LHON cases. Clinically, patients with visual loss from the 3 primary LHON mutations differ only in their propensity for visual recovery—patients with the 14484 mutation have a far greater chance of spontaneous recovery of vision (up to 70% of cases) than those patients with the 11778 or 3460 mutations (as low as 4% of cases).

The understanding of the genetic basis of LHON and the availability of molecular diagnosis on individual patients has allowed us to make a definitive diagnosis of this disorder even in patients without a family history of visual loss. However, we still do not know the exact location of the initial pathology within the optic nerve, the pathophysiology of optic nerve dysfunction, the explanation of the disease's peculiar timing and focal pathology, nor the determinants of expression. Indeed, the majority of patients who harbor a LHON mtDNA mutation will never express visual loss. Furthermore, the male predominance in this disorder cannot be explained by maternal inheritance and has recently been linked to a probable disease-modifying factor on the X chromosome. Environmental factors, both internal and external, may play a role in expression. Systemic illnesses, nutritional deficiencies, medications, or toxins that stress or directly inhibit mitochondrial metabolism could conceivably initiate or increase phenotypic expression of LHON. Although one large case-control study of sibships failed to confirm a role for tobacco and alcohol use as precipitants of visual loss, other studies have suggested that tobacco use may be more prevalent among those individuals who have lost vision from LHON.

The relatively easy access to laboratory testing for the 3 primary LHON mutations on blood samples allows us to consider the diagnosis of LHON not only in typical cases such as the one presented above, but also in any unusual or unexplained case of bilateral optic neuropathy. I would most certainly screen this young man for the primary LHON mutations. However, if his brother has already been tested and proved positive for a LHON mutation, there is no reason to confirm this on the patient or on his maternal relatives because all maternally related family members will have the mutation. I would certainly proceed with the planned MRI; although other causes of his optic neuropathy are far less likely, they have very different management implications. I would also obtain an electrocardiogram to screen for cardiac conduction defects.

Attempts to treat or prevent the acute phase of LHON visual loss with systemic or topical medications or vitamin supplementation have to date proven ineffective. There are anecdotal reports of improvement in vision with idebenone (a synthetic analog of Coenzyme Q10), but the possibility of spontaneous recovery, especially in young patients with the 14484 mutation, makes much of this literature inconclusive. Although some physicians will place these patients on "cocktails" of vitamins, especially those with purported antioxidant actions, I have not been impressed with any positive results. I most certainly recommend cessation of smoking, as I would anyway for general health reasons, but I only advise against excessive alcohol use. An assessment by a low-vision specialist may be helpful, especially given that a fair amount of peripheral vision may be retained.

The importance of genetic counseling of patients with LHON and their families cannot be overstated. The prognosis for visual recovery should be communicated based on the specific mutation harbored. Most importantly, it should be explained to this patient and his brother that neither of them can pass this disease to their children. However, all their female maternal relatives, whether affected with visual loss or not, will pass on the mutation, and hence the risk of visual loss, to all of their offspring.

Summary

* LHON is a clinical diagnosis confirmed by mitochondrial genetic testing.

* Attempts to treat or prevent the acute phase of LHON visual loss with systemic or topical medications or vitamin supplementation have to date proven ineffective.
* Recommend cessation of smoking and excessive alcohol use.
* The prognosis for visual recovery should be communicated based on the specific mitochondrial DNA mutation.

Bibliography

Man PYW, Turnbull DM, Chinnery PF. Leber hereditary optic neuropathy. *J Med Genet.* 2002;39:162-169.

Newman NJ. Hereditary optic neuropathies: from the mitochondria to the optic nerve. *Am J Ophthalmol.* 2005; 140(3):517-523.

Newman NJ. Hereditary optic neuropathies. In: Miller NR, Newman NJ, Biousse V, Kerrison JB, eds. *Walsh & Hoyt's Clinical Neuro-Ophthalmology.* 6th ed. Philadelphia, PA: Lippincott Williams & Wilkins; 2005:465-501.

Riordan-Eva P, Sanders MD, Govan GG, Sweeney MG, Da Costa J, Harding AE. The clinical features of Leber's hereditary optic neuropathy defined by the presence of a pathogenic mitochondrial DNA mutation. *Brain.* 1995;118:319-337.

How Do I Manage an Orbital Apex Syndrome?

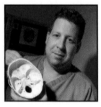

Roger E. Turbin, MD, FACS

A 35-year-old diabetic woman with a history of diabetic ketoacidosis (DKA) presents with new onset painful ophthalmoplegia and loss of vision in her right eye. There might be a bit of proptosis as well. What should I be worried about and how soon does she need to be seen?

The development of ophthalmoplegia and visual loss in a diabetic patient with keto-acidosis (DKA) is a neuro-ophthalmic emergency. It should be assumed to be due to a life-threatening invasive fungal infection until proven otherwise. Although such a patient may "walk into my office," I more frequently encounter this scenario in patients already hospitalized with DKA or suffering other immunosuppressive comorbid conditions, including cancer, chemotherapeutic treatment, long-term corticosteroid and broad-spectrum antibiotic therapy, chronic renal dialysis, and solid organ or bone marrow transplantation.

Accurate diagnosis begins with clinical localization, although the disease process may have already extended beyond ophthalmic and orbital structures to involve the cavernous sinus, paranasal sinuses, or cerebrovascular structures. Orbital apex syndrome (OAS) denotes involvement of the optic nerve in addition to some or all of the cranial nerves within the cavernous sinus/superior orbital fissure (III, IV, V, VI). Indeed, there is a lengthy differential diagnosis (Table 49-1) that will require confirmatory neuroimaging, laboratory support, and often histopathologic documentation.

My urgent ophthalmic examination includes an assessment of pupillary function (a surrogate for visual acuity or visual field if the patient is obtunded), assessment of proptosis and orbital congestion, motility analysis (III, IV, VI palsy versus motility

---

Table 49-1
Differential Diagnosis of Orbital Apex Syndrome

Inflammatory/Vasculitic
- Giant cell arteritis, polyarteritis nodosa, Churg Strauss, thyroid-associated orbitopathy, sarcoid, Wegener's, nonspecific orbital inflammation (pseudotumor)

Infectious
- Fungal (invasive, allergic), bacterial, viral, *Spirochete*

Neoplastic
- Benign
    - Contiguous structure (meningioma, pituitary, sinus, mucocele)
    - Neural (pituitary, meningioma, nerve and nerve sheath)
- Malignant
    - Primary malignancy
    - Contiguous structures (sinus carcinoma)
    - Metastatic
    - Hematologic

Vascular
- Aneurysmal, thrombosis, dural/carotid fistula, hypercoaguability state

Traumatic

Iatrogenic

Adapted from Yeh S, Foroozan R. Orbital apex syndrome. *Curr Opin Ophthalmol.* 2004;15:490-498.

---

disturbance due to congestion of the extraocular muscles), funduscopic examination (optic nerve and retinal perfusion, choroidal folds, cherry red macular spot), and other neurologic symptoms (including sympathetic dysfunction). I always assess trigeminal nerve function (corneal anesthesia, facial numbness) as areas of numbness (V1) signify extension to the cavernous sinus or beyond (V2, V3), as well as facial nerve and lower cranial nerve function. In addition, a direct visual inspection of the nasal and oropharyngeal mucosa, including soft and hard palate, is performed immediately to detect areas of necrosis. An emergent ear, nose, and throat (ENT) consultation must be obtained for endoscopic examination of the paranasal sinuses (Figure 49-1). Facial and endoscopic abnormalities are documented photographically for serial examination during follow-up.

I hospitalize or utilize the emergency room to coordinate ENT, neurosurgical, neurologic, medical, and infectious disease service consultations as well as emergent neuroimaging to include contrast-enhanced studies of the head and orbit. Both magnetic resonance imaging (MRI) and computed tomography (CT) are useful and provide adjunctive information for surgical planning, with MRI providing more soft tissue detail and CT providing detail of bone anatomy. Frequently we obtain both studies, and may

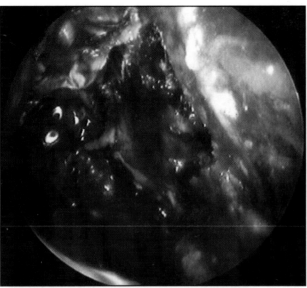

Figure 49-1. Endoscopic photograph of necrotic middle turbinate and ethmoid mucosa in a patient with biopsy-proven *Rhizopus* (*Mucor*). Initial intraoperative tissue analysis was suggestive of *Aspergillus nigrans.*

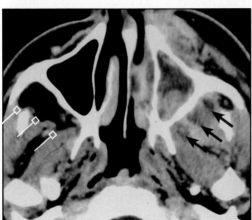

Figure 49-2. Contrast-enhanced axial CT scan shows loss of the normal fat plane behind the left maxillary sinus in the region of the pterygopalatine fossa (arrows) despite apparently intact bone in a patient with biopsy-proven *Rhizopus.* Compare this area to the normal black signal of the intact fat plane on the left of the figure (squares). There is also abnormal thickening and enhancement in the soft tissue of the face anterior to the maxillary sinus, as well as the left turbinate, maxillary sinus, and ethmoids (not shown).

supplement with vascular imaging (computed tomography angiography [CTA], magnetic resonance angiography [MRA], magnetic resonance venography [MRV], or cerebral angiography) as necessary. I pay special attention to the location of concurrent paranasal disease as most fungal infection spreads from the paranasal sinuses. I have found the destruction of the fat plane posterior to the maxillary sinus to be an indicator of invasive fungal disease and a sign that opacification of sinuses represents more than just incidental sinusitis (Figure 49-2). This radiographic sign may be missed or neglected unless specifically sought. Increased signal and enhancement in the orbital apex, extraocular muscles, and orbital tissues adjacent to sinus disease does not require bone destruction as spread may occur through intact bone via nutrient vascular foramina. In addition, unusual hypointense "black" signal on T2-weighted MRI images may serve as a hint that fungus is present due to signal change (paramagnetic susceptibility artifact) from the manganese in some species of fungal colonies (Figures 49-3 and 49-4).

Some clarification concerning taxonomy of invasive fungal infection is relevant. The term *mucormycosis* describes any fungal infection of the order *Mucorales*, which belongs

Figure 49-3. Contrast-enhanced coronal T1 fat-suppressed MRI of a patient with invasive *Aspergillus* shows diffuse areas of abnormal signal within all sinuses, turbinates, and right orbital apex (asterisk). Abnormal signal has extended beyond the plane of the skull base to involve the subfrontal extradural area (arrow) and both frontal lobes (squares).

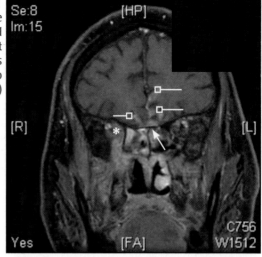

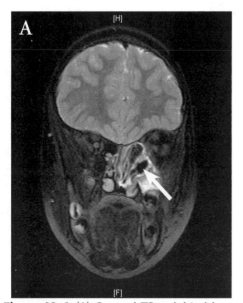

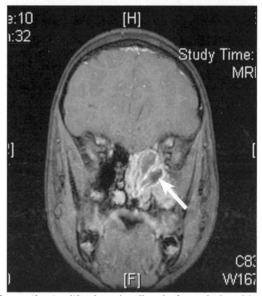

Figure 49-4. (A) Coronal T2-weighted image of a patient with chronic allergic fungal sinusitis from *Aspergillus fumigatus*. Paramagnetic susceptibility artifact in *Aspergillus* species can produce black signal (arrow) on T2 images simulating air. (B) T1 image of the same patient demonstrates that the area of *Aspergillus* infection is no longer black (arrow), and this discordance suggests fungal infection.

to the class *Zygomycetes* and may be termed *zygomycosis*. The terms *Rhizopus, Rhizomucor, Mucor,* and *Absidia* refer to the genus. *Rhizopus oryzae* is the predominant pathogenic species and accounts for 60% of all forms of mucormycosis and 90% of rhinocerebral forms. Aspergillosis refers to infection by *Deuteromycetes*, or imperfect fungi in which no sexual reproductive phase has been discovered. The 3 main pathogenic species are fumigatus, flavus, and niger. The early differentiation between the 2 most frequent invasive fungal pathogens, *Aspergillus* and *Zygomycetes*, has become increasingly important given the trend toward first line use of non-amphotericin B therapies with disparate fungal

Table 49-2
Broad Spectrum or Species-Directed Systemic Angifungal Therapy

Infection	Drug	Dosage/Duration	Alternatives
Aspergillosis	Voriconazole	6 mg/kg IV q12h x 1d, then 4 mg/kg IV bid or 200 to 300 mg PO bid >10 wks	
OR			
	Amphotericin B	1 to 1.5 mg/kg/d IV	Posaconazole 200 mg PO tid to qid
			Itraconazole 200 mg PO tid x 3d followed by 200 mg PO bid
			Caspofungin 70 mg IV x 1d, then 50 mg IV 1x/d
Zygomycosis	Amphotericin B	1 to 1.5 mg/kg/d IV	Posaconazole, 15 to 200 mg PO qid x 6 to 10 wks

We recommend that the above dosages be confirmed with your local infectious disease or other specialist as specific dosages may be subject to change or variation over time

Adapted from Turbin RE, Khoobiar SA, Langer P, et al. Adjuvant therapy for invasive sino-orbital fungal infection. *J Neuroophthalmol.* 2002;22:178-179.

sensitivities (Table 49-2). In additional, a noninvasive allergic form of chronic fungal sinusitis in atopic individuals exists (predominantly *Aspergillus* species) that responds to debridement and corticosteroid therapy (see Figure 49-4). This distinction is critical since corticosteroids are contraindicated in invasive fungal disease.

Historically, patients developing invasive fungal infection at the orbital apex suffer severe morbidity and frequent mortality. Survival requires early diagnosis and immediate treatment. Experienced authors have discussed treating infected tissues as a "malignancy" with extirpation of all involved tissues. This results in exenteration or even more extensive deforming craniofacial resection in patients with other comorbid conditions. I have moved away from this paradigm, utilizing surgery as an early diagnostic modality with a more limited resection of tissue that is ischemic or necrotic. In addition to broad spectrum or species-directed systemic angifungal therapy (see Table 49-2), it is my standard to use adjuvant direct antifungal application which I will discuss below. It has been my experience that despite standard textbook discussions citing that pathogens are easily differ iated based on microscopic morphology, the thinner, septate, acute branching angled *Aspergillus hyphae* will swell with frozen preparation and frequently be misinterpreted as *Mucor* or vice-versa (see Figure 49-1). This distinction is critical in order to begin appropriate therapy.

I consider surgical and systemic antifungal treatment supportive therapy until the primary immunosuppressive state can be reversed. Of note, the topical local application of amphotericin B discussed next may not represent Food and Drug Administration "approved" uses. If the underlying immunosuppressive state is not reversed with aggressive therapy (eg, treatment of DKA), it is very difficult to halt disease progression. In addition, the pathologic local environment at the site of infection may preclude adequate local antibiotic delivery to necrotic tissue through affected blood vessels. In addition, in *Mucor* infections, local changes produce acidotic conditions that promote fungal proliferation even after systemic DKA is corrected.

I always irrigate the affected soft tissues and sinuses intraoperatively with a liter of 0.25 to 0.50 mg/cc amphotericin B prepared by the pharmacy for surgical irrigation. I also typically perform postoperative retrobulbar or peribulbar injection of 2 to 6 cc of amphotericin B at 2 mg/cc prepared for injection in a sterile hood. I have injected this preparation as frequently as daily or in alternate day regimen up to 6 to 8 applications without significant adverse affect. I will direct the retrobulbar needle into the affected areas, administer a test dose with blood pressure monitoring present, and consider a peribulbar lidocaine injection if trigeminal sensation remains intact. Some authors have advocated an indwelling orbital catheter for irrigation, but I have found the retrobulbar or peribulbar injection adequate. Theoretically, a catheter might decrease the chance of an intradural injection through the nerve sheath or an ocular perforation, but it adds the added risk of an indwelling orbital foreign body. I do leave a postoperative catheter in place to irrigate the sinuses, which may require preirrigation application of topical anesthetic spray.

Summary

* An orbital apex syndrome in a diabetic or immunocompromised patient may represent a life-threatening fungal infection, and remains the primary diagnosis of exclusion.

* High clinical suspicion and early diagnosis of fungal infection is required to prevent significant morbidity or mortality.

* Diagnosis and treatment requires coordination of a multi-specialty approach.

* Advances in systemic antifungal therapy provide new potential alternatives to nephrotoxic monotherapy with amphotericin B.

* In fungal rhino-sino-orbital infection, biopsy, limited debridement, and systemic antifungal administration coupled with adjuvant local antifungal therapy may provide an alternative to mutilating extirpative surgical procedures.

Bibliography

Treatment Guidelines from the Medical Letter. *Antifungal Drugs.* 2008;6(issue 65):1-8.

Turbin RE, Khoobiar SA, Langer P, et al. Adjuvant therapy for invasive sino-orbital fungal infection. *J Neuroophthalmol.* 2002;22:178-179.

Yeh S, Foroozan R. Orbital apex syndrome. *Curr Opin Ophthalmol.* 2004;15:490-498.

Supported in part by Research to Prevent Blindness, Inc, New York, NY; Fund for the New Jersey Blind, Newark, NJ; Lions Eye Research Foundation of New Jersey, Newark, NJ; The Eye Institute of New Jersey, Newark, NJ; and the Gene C. Coppa Memorial Fund, Newark, NJ.

Financial Disclosures

QUESTION 1

Mark Borchert, MD has no financial disclosures to report.

QUESTION 2

Neil R. Miller, MD has no financial disclosures to report.

QUESTION 3

Fiona Costello, MD has received advisory board or speakers' fees from TEVA Neurosciences, Serono Biogen Idec, and Bayer in the past 12 months. She also received research funding from the MS Society of Canada and Neuroscience Canada.

QUESTION 4

Eric Eggenberger, DO, MSEpi receives unrestricted grants, research, and/or speaking support from Biogen, Teva, Bayer, and Serono.

QUESTION 5

Melissa W. Ko, MD has no financial disclosures to report.
Steven L. Galetta, MD has received speaking honorarium from BigoenIdec.

QUESTION 6

Rod Foroozan, MD has no financial disclosures to report.

QUESTION 7

M. Tariq Bhatti, MD has no financial disclosures to report.

QUESTION 8

Alfredo A. Sadun, MD, PhD has no financial disclosures to report.

QUESTION 9

Jacqueline A. Leavitt, MD has no financial disclosures to report.

QUESTION 10

Nicholas J. Volpe, MD has no financial disclosures to report.
Jennifer K. Hall, MD has no financial disclosures to report.

QUESTION 11

Michael Wall, MD has no financial disclosures to report.

QUESTION 12

Deborah I. Friedman, MD, FAAN has no financial disclosures to report.

QUESTION 13

Victoria S. Pelak, MD has no financial disclosures to report.
Drew Dixon, MD has no financial disclosures to report.

QUESTION 14

Christopher C. Glisson, DO has no financial disclosures to report.
David I. Kaufman, DO has no financial disclosures to report.

QUESTION 15

Laura J. Balcer, MD, MSCE has no financial disclosures to report.
Raymond Price, MD has no financial disclosures to report.

QUESTION 16

Pamela S. Chavis, MD has no financial disclosures to report.
Peter Savino, MD has no financial disclosures to report.

QUESTION 17

James A. Garrity, MD has no financial disclosure to report.

QUESTION 18

Steven E. Feldon, MD, MBA received an unrestricted grant from Research to Prevent Blindness, P.I.

QUESTION 19

Kimberly Cockerham, MD has no financial disclosure to report.

QUESTION 20

Janet C. Rucker, MD has no financial disclosure to report.

QUESTION 21

Sophia M. Chung, MD has no financial disclosure to report.

QUESTION 22

Brian R. Younge, MD has no financial disclosure to report.

QUESTION 23

Valérie Biousse, MD has no financial disclosure to report.

QUESTION 24

Randy Kardon, MD, PhD is a consultant with Ovation Pharmaceutical and Boehringer-Ingelheim Pharmaceuticals. He also receives royalties for book and pictures used in various textbooks co-authored in 1979, *Tissues and Organs: A Text-Atlas of Scanning Electron Microscopy.*

QUESTION 25

Aki Kawasaki, MD has no financial disclosure to report.

QUESTION 26

Julie Falardeau, MD, FRCSC received honorarium as a consultant for Ovation Pharmaceutical.

QUESTION 27

Swaraj Bose, MD has no financial disclosure to report.

QUESTION 28

Kathleen B. Digre, MD has no financial disclosure to report.

QUESTION 29

Karl C. Golnik, MD, MEd has no financial disclosure to report.

QUESTION 30

Grant T. Liu, MD has no financial disclosure to report.
Madhura A. Tamhankar, MD has no financial disclosure to report.

QUESTION 31

Steve Newman, MD has no financial disclosure to report.

QUESTION 32

James J. Corbett, MD has no financial disclosure to report.

QUESTION 33

Wayne T. Cornblath, MD has no financial disclosure to report.

QUESTION 34

Rosa Ana Tang, MD, MPH is on the speaker's bureau for Bayer.

QUESTION 35

Byron L. Lam, MD has no financial disclosure to report.

QUESTION 36

Jonathan C. Horton, MD, PhD has no financial disclosure to report.

QUESTION 37

Gautam R. Mirchandani, MD has no financial disclosure to report.
Jeffrey Odel, MD has no financial disclosure to report.
Sang-Rog Oh, MD has no financial disclosure to report.

QUESTION 38

Michael S. Vaphiades, DO has no financial disclosure to report.

QUESTION 39

Thomas J. Carlow, MD has no financial disclosure to report.

QUESTION 40

Matthew J. Thurtell, MBBS, FRACP has no financial disclosure to report.
Robert L. Tomsak, MD, PhD has no financial disclosure to report.

QUESTION 41

Steven R. Hamilton, MD has no financial disclosure to report.

QUESTION 42

Greg Kosmorsky, DO has no financial disclosure to report.

QUESTION 43

Timothy J McCulley, MD has no financial disclosure to report.
Thomas N Hwang, MD, PhD has no financial disclosure to report.

QUESTION 44

Michael S. Lee, MD has no financial disclosure to report.
Andrew R. Harrison, MD has no financial disclosure to report.

QUESTION 45

Robert L. Lesser, MD has no financial disclosure to report.

QUESTION 46

Robert H. Spector, MD has no financial disclosure to report.

QUESTION 47

Leah Levi, MBBS has no financial disclosure to report.

QUESTION 48

Nancy J. Newman, MD has no financial disclosure to report.

QUESTION 49

Roger E. Turbin, MD FACS has no financial disclosure to report.

INDEX

CURBSIDE
Consultation

The exciting and unique Curbside Consultation Series is designed to effectively provide ophthalmologists with practical, to the point, evidence based answers to the questions most frequently asked during informal consultations between colleagues.

Each specialized book included in the Curbside Consultation Series offers quick access to current medical information with the ease and convenience of a conversation. Expert consultants who are recognized leaders in their fields provide their advice, preferences, and opinions to answer the tricky questions that require ophthalmologists to practice the "art" of medicine.

Written with a similar reader-friendly Q and A format and including images, diagrams, and references, each book in the Curbside Consultation Series will serve as a solid, go-to reference for practicing ophthalmologists and residents alike.

Series Editor: David F. Chang, MD

Curbside Consultation in Cataract Surgery: 49 Clinical Questions
David F. Chang, MD

Curbside Consultation in Cornea and External Disease: 49 Clinical Questions
Eduardo C. Alfonso, MD

Curbside Consultation in Glaucoma: 49 Clinical Questions
Dale K. Heuer, MD

Curbside Consultation in Neuro-Ophthalmology: 49 Clinical Questions
Andrew G. Lee, MD

Curbside Consultation in Refractive Surgery: 49 Clinical Questions
Eric D. Donnenfeld, MD

Curbside Consultation of the Retina: 49 Clinical Questions
Sharon Fekrat, MD

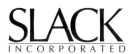